Intermittent Fasting

For Women Over 50:

Back to Youth

The complete Anti-Aging Plan to Prevent

Inflammation, Boost your Metabolism, Detox your

body and Lose Weight Naturally

Jennifer Young

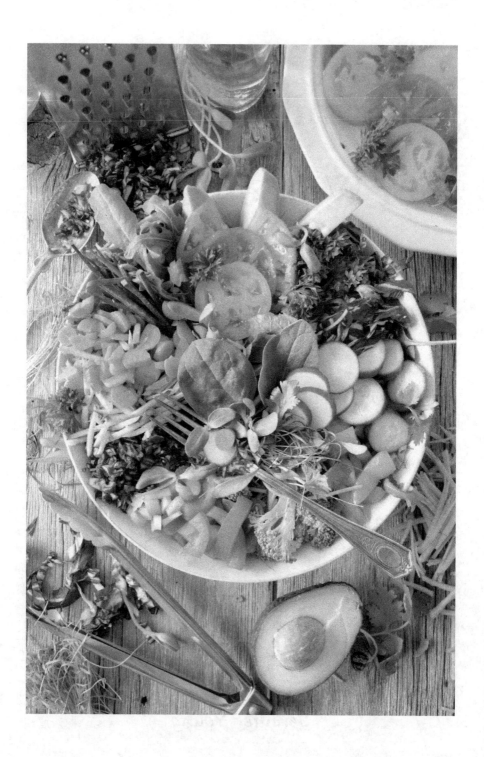

Table of contents

INTRODUCTION 7

WHAT IS MENOPAUSE? 10

CAUSES OF WEIGHT GAIN IN MENOPAUSE................................... 14

INTERMITTENT FASTING: WHAT IS IT, AND HOW DOES IT WORK?................... 17

THE PROVEN BENEFITS OF INTERMITTENT FASTING AFTER 50 21

WHY DOES INTERMITTENT FASTING HELP TO PROMOTE WEIGHT LOSS? 24

IS INTERMITTENT FASTING SAFE FOR EVERYONE?........................... 26

WHO SHOULD AVOID INTERMITTENT FASTING? 31

WHAT DOES SCIENCE SAY? THE MUST-KNOW EFFECTS OF INTERMITTENT FASTING ON HEALTH AND AGING 32

WHY THE RIGHT MINDSET IS MORE IMPORTANT THAN DIET.......................... 38

    RULE 1: MAKE A PLAN..42
    RULE 2: VALUATE EVERY SMALL OR LARGE GOAL YOU REACH 43
    RULE 3: HAVE A FOCUS 43

WHICH TYPE OF INTERMITTENT FASTING SHOULD YOU CHOOSE ACCORDING TO YOUR BODY.. 46

A DAY IN THE LIFE OF IF 49

HOW TO MAXIMIZE YOUR INTERMITTENT FASTING RESULTS......................... 51

COMMON INTERMITTENT FASTING MISTAKES TO AVOID 53

NUTRITION BASICS: WHAT ARE MACRONUTRIENTS AND MICRONUTRIENTS... 56

THE BEST NUTRIENTS AND VITAMINS AFTER 50 62

A PROTOCOL FOR 16:8 INTERMITTENT FASTING 72

A PROTOCOL FOR 24-HOUR INTERMITTENT FASTING....................... 74

OTHER TYPES OF INTERMITTENT FASTING 75

HOW TO GET STARTED WITH INTERMITTENT FASTING.................................. 77

WHAT CAN YOU EAT AND DRINK WHILE INTERMITTENT FASTING.................. 79

UNHEALTHY FOODS YOU SHOULD REMOVE FROM YOUR DIET....................... 81

ANTI-AGING SUPERFOODS 84

HOW TO TRACK YOUR NUTRITION INTAKE EASILY AND EFFECTIVELY 93

INCORPORATING EXERCISE INTO YOUR FASTING REGIME 97

THE FINAL HEALTHY LIFESTYLE: HOW LOSING WEIGHT TRIGGERS A CASCADE OF HEALTH BENEFITS... 100

FAQ.. 104

CONCLUSION... 108

Introduction

There is no denying it. Obesity has reached epidemic proportions and is widespread in most Western countries. It begins to spread in Asia, and people become more and more overweight and obese. It is almost impossible to hide the news and discussion about the obesity epidemic that takes lives and breaks the quality of life worldwide. It is in papers, on television, and blogged on the internet almost constantly. If this is not enough, unless you are blind, it is challenging to browse any big city or small-town streets and not see the final product of this first-hand epidemic. The truth is that people grow, and it's a real health crisis that only a fool could ignore. There are many reasons here are only the most blinding ... Many people eat far too often, too often. It is a complicated truth that cannot be escaped. The human body has not been designed by nature to eat as often as most people do it. Our bodies are machines designed for survival.

Delete a little hunger from our lives, and we will pack on the fat and pack it at the speed of lightning—a widespread avoidance of the exercise. After overeating, the next huge problem is exercised. People have fewer physical jobs, and social lives revolve around digital rather than physics, once again our body of what they have been designed for: run, lift, hunting, and playing. The least muscular we wear less our metabolism, which means even more fat is packaged. Do you see a developing model?

The lack of sleep quality

The first two obesity builders first contributed to the third. A bad diet and lack of exercise offer a quick lane for a damaged sleep pattern shown in further research that can also be calculated to injure the metabolism and pack fat. A night without sleep throws and turns quickly, the same as the flab's bad spare tire at the waist.

Medicines and drugs

Medicines and drugs that come with the growing medical community are the side effects of all these drugs, including weight and lethargy. A culture that is approaching health more naturally and holistic has avoided chiefly this problem and can also avoid health problems related to the accompanying obesity. Our society hasn't known this yet. These are only a few of many reasons for obesity outbreaks spread so fast and deadly. There are many more, believe me. The question stands: what can we do? How can we turn off the wave of obesity? The answer is, of course, diet and sports. There are many diverse ideas about both, some good and evil. This complete guide offers what I feel may be the perfect solution for most people's struggles wearing a fat. This is quite simple and packed with strength, in line with common nature and sense. The most crucial thing works and works almost like magic.

So, why did this happen? Why are there more overweight people than before? There are several reasons for this. The first reason is our diet. Today too many people are addicted to Junk Food, processed food, white flour products, etc. All of these meals cause blood sugar levels to surge, and this, in turn, causes fat storage and insulin insurgents. Stable lifestyles are another reason. With coming of technology, many manual tasks are more accessible and less demanding. Need to go to a supermarket which is a 20-minute walk away? Get a car instead of walking. Need to go up to level 3 in your office building? Take the elevator, not a ladder. All activities that burn calories are avoided and replaced with a more accessible alternative. As a result, people are far more vulnerable to gaining weight. Much easier to watch TV with a bag of potato chips rather than running. It's much easier to drink a bottle of processed apple juice than eating raw apples. It's all this little action that is important. In the US, Junk Food is often cheaper than healthy and nutritious food to worsen the situation. Low-income families can easily buy junk food but struggle to pay for "authentic food." This is one reason why obesity affects more low-income families. There is one cure to reverse weight gain and obesity. It is powerful that people can lose weight even on the Junk Food diet only by adopting this method. This is called intermittent fasting. We will call it as if starting now to make everything easier. Unlike diets such as the Atkins diet or lemonade diet, intermittent fasting is a unique method that does not regard its own food with food consumed. It's more focused on timing. If you strive to lose weight or if you have an appetite that you cannot control, fasting intermittently is your answer. If you try to see your stomach but can't burn the last layer of fat on your stomach, fasting intermittent has your name written on it. This is truly one of the most influential and extraordinary methods to lose weight.

Why is Intermittent Fasting so Popular?

Obesity is an increasing problem. So, it's not a surprise that so many people are looking for a better way to lose weight. Traditional diets that limit calories often fail to work for many people. It's hard to follow this type of diet in the long run. This often leads to the Yo-yo diet - the endless cycle of weight loss and profit. This often results in mental health problems, but it can also cause more overall weight gain. So, many people have searched for a long-term diet. Intermittent fasting is one of these diets— more than lifestyle changes than eating plans, different from the regular diet. Many intermittent fasting followers feel easy to follow for a long time. Even better, this helps them lose weight effectively. However, this type of eating plan offers benefits from weight loss. Many people believe that it can provide health benefits. Some of the services are even said to stretch further; some say it makes them more focused and productive. As a result, they become more successful at work. The latest stories in the Media CEO claim their successes all go down to intermittent fasting. However, the benefit does not stop there. There is evidence to show that intermittent fasting helps health in other ways too. It also improves blood sugar levels and immunity.

This can improve brain function, reduce inflammation, and repair cells in the body as well. With all this in mind, it's easy to see why this diet is becoming more popular. Here, we will look at why Intermittent fasting serves to increase weight loss. We will check the benefits of this lifestyle change, and we will show you how to start with this diet protocol. Also called the Feast and Famine Diet, it can change your life for the better. You will know everything about Intermittent Fasting, everything on how to make it work and get the lean and healthy body of your dreams. Get ready. This is going to be a blast!

What is Menopause?

The menopausal term refers to the process that occurs naturally in women due to aging. It produces the absence of menstrual periods and the inability to get pregnant. Usually, menopause occurs between ages 45 and 55. This is a new phase in women's lives involving several physical and emotional changes. During menopause, women's estrogen levels decrease naturally. This can lead to menopausal symptoms, which vary and can be light to severe. Sometimes, some women may experience initial menopause (or premature), which occurred before 40 years.

Because this is a physiological condition in a woman's body, which is part of the natural aging process, the prognosis is based on everyone's symptoms. It will depend on the timeliness of intervention, the age where it occurs, and the patient's health status. Symptoms of menopause can start months or years before the termination of total menstruation and usually lasts around four years after the end of the period. The most common symptoms include:

- Hot flashes
- Vaginal dryness
- Difficulty sleeping
- Low morale
- Anxiety
- Loss of libido
- Night sweats
- Difficulty concentrating

Premenopause and menopause: what are they?

You know that your body is influenced by your activities and hormone cycles. This reality does not change even when you face menopause. Menopause starts a year after your last period. On average, it happened between the ages of forty-five fifty-five. The transition does not occur sharply and suddenly; you arrive at this stage by undergoing premenopausal, also known as climactically. Another delicate moment that every woman must be prepared for. This is a variable period - can last from two to ten years - before the last menstruation. One-third of the life of a woman is spent appropriately in premenopausal and menopause. That's why you must immediately take a healthy, healthy, and peaceful approach. Start with food; your welfare must pass through the power of food. To determine a correct diagnosis of menopause, it is necessary to consult with your doctor, who will be able to set possible therapy. It may be required to carry out specific examinations such as pap-test and mammography to exclude the existence of pathology, to monitor the level of female hormones, and assess bone mineral density. When you get older, it changes your sex hormones, and your ovaries don't produce as much estrogen as they use. This means that ovules are no longer released from ovaries. Menopause is a natural process of aging for women but sometimes it occurs earlier than expected, without a definite cause. In some cases, menopause can be caused by therapeutic treatments, such as treatment for breast cancer (for example, chemotherapy or radiation therapy). The elimination of ovarian surgery can also cause menopause.

Menopause is a stage in women's development and cannot be prevented. What can be done is consider specific treatments to reduce the risk of long-term problems such as osteoporosis and heart disease. With the onset of menopause or during the premenopausal period, hormone levels down, their protective effects are reduced, and it becomes easier to stack the excess pounds. However, the modification of hormonal currents is not the only obstacle that stands in front of the woman who wants to fit. There are several factors that, put together, make it difficult for those who have entered menopause to find or regain their ideal forms (which may no longer be a pre-menopause period). During the menopausal phase, it can be more challenging to lose weight and complicated to avoid weight. Why is it so complicated to lose weight during menopause and maintain the ideal weight? Basically, there are three leading causes:

- Deceleration of basal metabolism, which sided with the accumulation of fat in the hip, thighs, and stomach;
- Hormonal change (Estrogen and Progesterone Drop);
- Increased cortisol levels (stress hormones) caused by stress, the state of anxiety and depression, promotes the accumulation of abdominal fat.

If menopause symptoms occur before 45 years, it is recommended to consult your family doctor and discuss your ongoing symptoms. Doctor can request a blood test to determine whether your symptoms are indeed related to menopause. Blood tests can also be asked for patients under the age of 40 if doctor, after symptom evaluation, wants to confirm the suspicion of early menopause.

So, your body is changing. You have frequent hot flashes, your cycle is unstable, and your mood; do you feel like you don't recognize yourself anymore and that things are getting out of hand? You will go through Premenopause. This is the transition period; it's true, but you don't think it comes down to a fast and smooth transition.

Unfortunately, premenopausal can last for years and really bring many changes in your life. That's why you need to realize it immediately and take action with all the tools you can to find yourself, your balance, and continue your life happily. Let's see what happens in this phase and how to set it thanks to the proper diet. Basal metabolic rate is represented by the number of calories consumed by our body when resting. The physiological slowdown in the vital function that occurs with the arrival of menopause leads the body to consume fewer calories. If you continue eating as you did before menopause, therefore, you might gain weight without knowing the reason. After a certain age, the muscle mass starts to decline, and the muscles tend to be hypertrophic. If you don't practice sports, your body will become less and less fast, and your weight will increase. Among other causes of difficulty in losing weight, or excess weight in menopause there may be:

- slowing of thyroid activity;
- unhealthy lifestyles
- unhealthy diet;
- sedentariness;
- insomnia, anxiety, and depression

For this reason, it is essential to adapt your habits and lifestyle to the new needs of your body, which is going through a moment of fragility, trying to keep your body weight under control.

Why is it difficult to lose weight after the age of 40?

Do you experience this transition now and struggle with weight gain? Your diet is the same as that always happens, but you gain weight. The explanation lies in your new hormone balance. The level of sex hormone, progesterone, and estrogen, decreases, and at the same time, androgens tend to increase. These hormones affect sleep, calcium loss in your bones, assimilate nutrition, and other symptoms. Knowing your hormonal rhythm is the starting point to understand your metabolism and regain a harmonious body.

What should be done to act on menopausal symptoms? We just saw that hormones found a different balance; this involves gradual modification of your dietary needs. The two main objectives are: to ward off a digestive slowdown and stimulate the removal of toxins. To facing the transition to premenopausal and menopause in a possible peaceful way, the right food, combined in the right way, brings great benefits.

Causes of Weight Gain in Menopause

According to the latest surveys, more than 7 of the 10 women complain of weight gain with menopausal arrivals. The tendency to get excess pounds, with the distribution that is not harmonious in body, is widespread. "But it is possible to control weight, with a few simple steps - said many experts - and not to gain weight also important because body fat increases the risk of many diseases." The Increased weight is the consequence of hormonal and metabolic changes that accompany this period.

Women have by constitution a higher total amount of body fat than men. The average percentage of body fat in a normal-weight woman is actually like an overweight man. This difference has been present at birth and becomes more felt at puberty: weight gain is mainly due to increased lean body mass in men and a group of fat in women. Also, the different types and distribution of fats between men and women: men tend to accumulate more visceral fats, especially at the abdominal level, and are more susceptible to central obesity; However, women before menopause tend to deposit more fat in subcutaneous tissue, especially at the gluteal-femoral level and more susceptible to peripheral obesity. After menopause, this peculiarity is lost to support the deposition of visceral and stomach fat. Increasing weight in menopause is inevitable? When the menstrual cycle disappears, the decline in estrogen production and hormone changes can be reflected throughout the body, affecting metabolism and mood. Among the typical symptoms of menopause, it is possible to find a sudden hot flash, skin drought along with reducing firmness and elasticity of the skin, excessive night sweat, vaginal dryness, concentration, and memory problems.

Among changes are usually related to the menopausal period. There is also a weight change, but this does not have to happen: menopause does not mean cursing to gain weight. However, throughout a woman's life, even in pre-menopause, body changes because we face various periods and stages. Following are the things you need to know about why you gain weight during menopause.

Scientific causes: how metabolism changes

The weight and change of the body during menopause, such as losing muscle tone and a less pleasant body feeling, have a significant relationship the with metabolism, decreasing with age.

What is the rate of basal metabolism? Called the basal metabolism level in English, the rate of basal metabolism (MB or BMR) shows the energy expenditure of an organism at rest, which is needed to maintain vital function during a state of awake, so the fundamental process is like digestion, respiration, blood circulation, and activities related to the nervous system. The value of basal metabolism, expressed in kilocalories (kcal), represents around 70% of the total energy expenditure in a day: it tends to decrease by 8% every ten years. According to research, the habit of physical training and diets rich in fiber and protein can positively affect the rate of basal metabolism, which must be calculated by considering an organism at rest, fasting for 12 hours.

The amount of fat on average between 20 and 60 years increases from 40 to 50%, even among women who maintain equal body weight. The percentage of abdominal obesity increases. In addition to the statistics, what is essential to do is a healthy and honest analysis of our life habits.

Why is it important to keep weight under control?

The problem is far beyond aesthetic aspects: it is scientifically documented that overweight is a risk factor for many chronic diseases like high blood pressure, dyslipidaemia (hypercholesterolemia), type II diabetes, heart, and cerebrovascular disease (heart attack, heart failure, Stroke), respiratory disease, liver and gallbladder, cancer (such as breast, ovarian, endometrium, and rectum) and osteoarthritis. "Belly Fat" in particular can be dangerous: actually, a close correlation has been shown between the accumulation of fat in the stomach and the risk of cardiovascular and diseases such as diabetes and cancer.

Women, who thank estrogen are protected from cardiovascular disease throughout their childbearing years, are exposed to very high-risk during menopause due to changes in the metabolism of fats and sugars and the presence of risk factors such as overweight, hypertension, and diabetes: so much so that these diseases are the main cause of death in women, even before breast cancer.

What are the parameters to be monitored?

There are two critical parameters to keep controlling your weight: body mass index (BMI) obtained by dividing weight by the square of the height. The value of BMI lower than 25 shows people who are average weight; from 25 to 30 one overweight; From 30 to 40 shows obesity and more than 40 forms of severe obesity. BMI is an estimated index because it does not consider the type of physical constitution, fat localization, and muscle mass.

Other values that need to be noted are waist circumference (measured at the height of navel), which is abdominal adipose network index connected with cardiovascular disease risk and must not exceed 31 ½ inches. Neuroscience study of neuroplasticity shows that physical activity, and active lifestyle habits, are natural drugs for the body and have regenerative effects on the brain because they contribute to creating new neuron connections by strengthening existing networks. However, research shows that often female groups in menopausal periods show less physical activity than others. Of course, some factors can be attributed to everyday life: Often, a woman aged between 50 and 60 years still devotes a few hours a day to work; Other times are usually dedicated to home care, cleaning, and cooking, in addition to the role of grandma, often increasingly demanding. People don't have time for themselves and delay undefended activities that look excessive, as swimming or take a walk. Usually, the hormone changes produce storms that reflect the mood, accentuate stress and anger, consequences for nervous hunger, and the tendency to fill emotional holes. Also, it is crucial to consider that we often continue to feed the body in the same way we have used all our lives. But in the meantime, body changes! The type of diet and eating habits you have had no longer adequate for your needs now, which is why it is essential to take opportunity to deal with changes with consciousness, rather than living it, at the physical and psychological level.

Intermittent Fasting: What is it, and how does it work?

Intermittent fasting quickly became a popular choice among those who try to lose weight. However, this is also popular with many other people who also want to reap health benefits and health. So, what is intermittent fasting? Basically, intermittent fasting is a way of feeding rather than a regular diet. Standard diets focus on what to eat. Generally, diets focus on daily calorie counts and specific foods. This leads to dieters constantly thinking about what they are and aren't allowed to eat. Fatty and sweet food is completely prohibited. Commonly diets focus on vegetables, fruit, and low-fat, low-sugar food. Those who follow a classical diet often end up fantasizing about treats and snacks. While they can lose weight, they might struggle to stick to their eating plans in the long term. Intermittent fasting is different. This is a lifestyle than a diet. This involves a diet where you bike between fasting windows and eating. Unlike other diets, intermittent fasting doesn't focus on what you can eat. Instead, it focuses on when you have to eat.

Those who follow the steps of intermittent fasting enjoy more freedom than this eating style gives them. In fact, they have more choices concerning foods with which to feed themselves without guilt. Many people also find that this style fits better into their daily routine. However, exist some potential pitfalls when it comes to intermittent fasting for weight loss.

The Origins of Intermittent Fasting

There is no one particular place where intermittent fasting comes from. In fact, it is based on the traditional way we eat. In the past, foods were rare: if you wanted to eat, you had to hunt. In the days when you managed to find food or to track, it worked, there would be a party. If hunting were slim and there was no food, you wouldn't have eaten. This ancient situation will be similar to fasting. The only difference is that our ancestors didn't have much choice.

Because of this method of eating and fasting, our ancestors were rarely overweight. They also led much more active lives since there was no technology to assist them. So, we can assume a certain level that the human body instinctively adapts to fasting intermittently. We may have evolved technologically, but we are almost the same as our ancestors when it comes to our physiology. However, intermittent Fasting is a relatively new lifestyle choice. There are verses in the Bible and the Koran about fasting for religious purposes. Many religious people are still fast today for reasons of religion. Ramadhan is when Muslims do not eat from sunset to sunbathing.

Therefore, it is easy to see where the idea of intermittent fasting originated. Fasting was also practiced by ancient Greek civilizations. In many primitive cultures, fasting was considered an essential phase of many rituals. Fasting was also the basis of some political protests: for example, with Suffragettes during the early twentieth century. Fasting for therapeutic purposes was also a trend during the 1800s, used to cure many diseases and treat the poor. Carried out under an expert's supervision, this type of fast is adopted to treat many hypertension conditions to headaches. Each fasting is tailored to individual needs. It can be a day or up to three months. Although Fasting fell out of favour as new medications were developed, it has recently re-emerged. In recent years, the term "Intermittent Fasting" has been one of the most searched terms on online search engines. So, what should you know about it? Intermittent Fasting is the rage in health, fitness, and weight loss circles. Its ideas make it to publication and comprehensive practice. It's popular because it works!

A cyclical diet

As the name suggests, intermittent fasting is a cyclical diet that involves fasting followed by a period where you eat. The non-fasting period can vary depending on the type of fasting intermittently you do. There are several types of intermittent fasting. We will now highlight some popular and recommend the most accessible type to ensure you the best result.

Intermittent fasting can be broken down into 2 "windows."

- Fasting window

- Eating window

During the fasting window, you will not be allowed to consume any food. You can only drink water. No calories should be consumed during fasting window. During the eating period you will be allowed to eat and consume all your calories during this window. Intermittent fasting does not concern what you eat. The diet is secondary. What is important is that you must obey the fasting period. This is when the body will take advantage of fat energy stores. The fasting principle is when your stomach is empty, the body will not have food for fuel and will use fat stores for fuel. This is very important in burning fat. Many people struggle to lose weight because their insulin store is complete, and the body burns food as fuel. The body never gets the opportunity to access fat shops. As a result, even with exercise, changes look slow to come. Anyway, even if you have adopted intermittent fasting, you must try to do a calorie deficit to guarantee fat loss. If you are on a calorie deficit, and you combine it with intermittent fasting, your fat will melt faster than you have ever thought.

Let's analyze an example. If you have an 8-hour meal window and a 16-hour fasting window, you need to consume all your calories in 8 hours. The beauty of Intermittent Fasting is that your body will not go into "starvation mode" because you will be eating and consuming calories. You will only do it in a shorter time. So, assuming you finish all your calories during the 8 hours, about 3 to 4 hours after your last meal, the food you ate would have been digested. Some calories may have been used as fuel by your body. However, in this way, there are about 12 hours away to go before the next meal because you are in 16 hours. Your body will not have more food to use as fuel. That's when it will use insulin and fat stores for energy. It doesn't matter if you wake up or sleep; Your body will burn calories for all different body processes such as repairs and maintenance. These calories will come from stored fat. This is what makes Intermittent Fasting so fantastic. Like the Master Leonardo da Vinci said, "Simplicity is the ultimate sophistication."

Intermittent fasting is extremely simple in concept. It doesn't involve detoxification, low carbs, ketogenic dieting, etc. None of that is an issue. All you need to do is enjoy eating and fast... that's it. It doesn't get any simpler. Now let's look at how it came about.

Why do People Prefer Intermittent Fasting?

Unlike other diets, intermittent fasting allows those who follow this eating style to eat pretty much whatever they want. In fact, those on intermittent fasting can eat sweet or fatty foods or go out to eat without worrying about calorie counting. Those who follow intermittent fasting don't have to eat food they don't like. They don't need to feel like they are seizing the food they love. With that said, it's easy to see why this is a popular choice. Not only that, but intermittent fasting offers more benefits than other types of diets. Yes, indeed, it promotes rapid weight loss. However, it also helps you feel more focused and more productive, healthier, and more energetic. Given the many benefits this style of eating offers, it's no wonder people prefer it over regular diets.

The Proven Benefits of Intermittent Fasting after 50

There are several benefits that those who take part in the intermittent fasting style report. Here, we look closer to some of the most common ones.

Weight Loss

Generally, people who do intermittent fasting do so to lose weight quickly. There is evidence to show that this method of eating helps you to spill pounds faster. There are several reasons intermittent fasting helps a weight loss: it improves metabolic functions for faster fat burning. It also reduces the calories you consume in a day. By lowering insulin levels, increasing norepinephrine, and increasing growth hormone levels, intermittent fasting accelerating fat damage. Also, it facilitates the use of fat to produce energy for the body. Fasting for a short time has been shown to increase the rate of metabolism by 14%. This means you will burn more calories. As a result, intermittent fasting can help cause weight loss of up to 8% for 3-24 weeks. It's an impressive loss! Those who try it reporting a 7% reduction in waist circumference. This shows that intermittent fasting helps you lose visceral fat in the abdominal area. This most dangerous fat exposes to many diseases. Moreover, intermittent fasting minimizes the loss of muscle mass compared to other low-calorie diets.

Repairing Cells

When you fast, your body's cells begin the process of removing waste cells. This is known as "autophagy." Autophagy involves the damaged body cells. It also involves dysfunctional metabolization and damaged proteins that have built over time in cells. What are the benefits of autophagy? Well, experts believe that he offers protection from development of several diseases. This includes Alzheimer's disease and cancer. Therefore, if you follow the intermittent fasting regime, you can help protect yourself from infection. As a result, you can live longer and healthier.

Insulin Sensitivity

More people than ever before suffer from type 2 diabetes. This disease becomes more common because of increasing obesity. The main feature of diabetes is an increase in blood sugar levels due to insulin resistance. Intermittent fasting can reduce insulin. Consequently, blood sugar levels will be reduced. This will offer excellent protection from development of type 2 diabetes. Intermittent fasting has been shown to have the main benefit when it comes to insulin resistance. It can highly reduce the levels of sugar in the blood. During the recent studies of intermittent fasting with human participants, it was shown that blood sugar levels decreased by up to 5-6% during the fasting period. So, fasting insulin levels can reduce by as much as 30%. This shows that intermittent fasting can offer benefits to reduce the possibility of developing diabetes. Another research, conducted on lab mice, shows that intermittent fasting protects against damage to kidneys. This is a complication associated with diabetes. So, once again, it is shown that intermittent fasting is also a good choice for anyone who suffers from diabetes.

Enhanced Brain Function

When something is good for body, it's often good for your brain too. Intermittent fasting is known to increase some metabolic features. This is very important for good brain health. Intermittent fasting has been shown to reduce oxidative stress. It also reduces inflammation and lowers blood sugar levels. Not only that, but it also reduces insulin resistance. These are all critical factors in improving brain functions. Studies were done on mice lab also show that intermittent fasting can help increase new nerve cells' growth.

It also offers benefits when it comes to brain function. Meanwhile, it also increases the level of BDNF (brain-derived neurotrophic factor). This is a brain hormone, and if you are deficient in it, you may suffer from brain problems and depression. When you try intermittent fasting, you will have better protection than this problem. As an additional advantage, studies in animals have shown that intermittent fasting can protect against the damage to brain from stroke. All of this indicates that intermittent fasting offers many brain health benefits.

Decreased Inflammation

It is well known that oxidative stress is a critical factor in chronic diseases and aging. Oxidative stress involves free radicals, which are unstable molecules that react with other significant DNA and protein molecules. The result is damage to molecules that cause damage to the body. Several studies prove that intermittent fasting can help improve your body's ability to hold oxidative stress. Other studies show it can help fight inflammation which unfortunately is the cause of many common diseases.

Why Does Intermittent Fasting Help to Promote Weight Loss?

Although intermittent fasting offers many benefits, the biggest is weight loss. Most people who start this lifestyle hope to spill pounds and maintain a healthy weight. So, why does intermittent fast help promote weight loss? Here, we will see three main reasons.

Reduced Calorie Intake

The main reason that intermittent fasting helps increase weight loss is that you naturally eat less. When you only have a short meal window, you have fewer times to eat. Usually, you will lose at least one meal per day to accommodate this schedule. In this way, in each 24 hours you will consume fewer calories. As you know, you must maintain a calorie deficit to lose weight. Therefore, intermittent fasting helps you achieve your weight loss goal effectively. It is important to note that some people fail to lose weight when they do it quickly. This is because they don't reduce their calorie intake. During their meal window, they continue to eat as much as they have if they usually eat. Therefore, they do not have the calorie deficit needed to spill pounds. As long as you don't overeat during your meal window, you will automatically reduce your calorie intake.

Hormonal Changes Boost Metabolism

Our body stores as energy in body fat. If you do not eat, your body changes several things so that the stored energy can be accessible - these changes involve the activity of the nervous system. They also include significant changes in several critical hormones. These changes occur in metabolism when we are fasting: insulin increases whenever you eat. If you are fast, insulin level will decrease considerably. A lower insulin level facilitates fuel combustion. Human Growth Hormone skyrockets when you are quick. This can increase as much as five times its average level. Hormonal growth helps fat loss and muscle gain. Noradrenaline is sent by the nervous system to fat cells, and this causes them to break your body fat. The grease is transformed into free fatty acids. These are then burned to produce energy. Many people believe that if you are looking for your metabolism slows down. However, evidence shows that short-term fasting can increase fat burning. Two studies have fasting 48 hours increases metabolism up to 14%.

Reduced Insulin Levels Speed Fat Burning

You probably know about insulin because of its essential role for diabetics. People who suffer from diabetes must take insulin to maintain normal function. However, many people are not sure what insulin does in the body or even what it is. Insulin is a hormone produced by the pancreas. Its job is to change glucose (sugar) in the blood into energy. Cells then use that energy as a source of energy. Insulin also has another role to play in our body: it encourages fat storage. Insulin levels in body will increase every time you eat and decrease every time you fast. Lower insulin levels caused when you quickly can help prevent excess fat storage and help the body mobilize the stored fat. As a result, it can increase your fat loss and help you lose weight faster.

Is Intermittent Fasting Safe for Everyone?

You might want to start an intermittent fasting style, but you can be worried about security. However, not every diet is suitable for everyone. The critical factor in a safe and successful weight loss is to get enough nutrients. In fact, if you don't get enough minerals, vitamins, and proteins, you can get sick. With too few calories and eating patterns too tight, you might not get enough nutrients. This can cause you to have medical problems. Nothing is suitable for everyone and this applies to intermittent fasting too. So, for these reasons, I suggest you consult a doctor before embarking on any dietary path. Anyway, intermittent fasting is safe for most people. In fact, it will be beneficial.

Recent research has shown that many people who start intermittent fasting program experience health benefits as increased fat burning and higher metabolic rates. Their blood pressure, harmful cholesterol levels, blood sugar levels improved dramatically. If you are worried about fasting intermittently, you must eliminate your fear. If you think about it, everyone passes through the fasting period when they sleep. If you sleep for 8 hours, you will be in a condition of fasting. The reason many people do not enjoy the benefits of this fasting country is caused by the fact that most people sleep less than 8 hours. Next, people eat before going to bed. So, when they sleep, the food is being digested. The body did not get the chance to be in a state of fasting too long. When they wake up, they have breakfast and start eating all day. There is very little time for body to tap into its fat stores. People with gastric problems, diabetes, etc. Must consult a doctor before starting the intermittent fasting program. Your doctor will be the best person to tell you if you can follow intermittent fasting. The good news is that intermittent fasting seems to be a safe method for most people. However, there are some cases where intermittent fasting should be avoided.

Could Intermittent Fasting Trigger an Eating Disorder?

Most people find many benefits and get splendid results in following a regimen of intermittent fasting. However, some people will not see well in this lifestyle. Some people have a natural tendency to develop irregular eating behaviour. These people may need to avoid intermittent fasting if it triggers an eating disorder.

It's therefore vital to recognize if intermittent fasting has strayed into patterns of disordered eating. There are several symptoms to look for:

- You have anxiety about eating food.
- You're feeling extremely tired.
- You're experiencing menstrual changes, mood swings, and problems are sleeping.

For those who have genetic tendencies for irregular diet, intermittent fasting can be dangerous. This is because there is a focus on not eating. Most diets focus on lowering your calorie intake by eating low-calorie foods. Intermittent fasting minimizes your calorie intake by avoiding eating during a specific period. This can lead you to ignore the signal of hunger from your body. Also, for someone with a tendency to develop eating disorders, you may become afraid of food due to Intermittent fasting. This is because you can start associating avoiding food by losing weight. Your brain may begin to reward you for not eating and develop a fear of eating time. Some people find that Intermittent fasting dieting causes them to binge eat. When they are in their meal window, they end up indulging in high-calorie food. This mimic eating disorder behaviour. Therefore, it is essential to be highly aware of any possible signs that your fasting is turning into an eating disorder.

What are the Side Effects of Intermittent Fasting?

Intermittent fasting offers many benefits but has side effects as well. These may affect each individual differently. Some effects that you might experience include:

- Feel angry, irritable, and upset because of hunger

- Experience brain mist or excessive fatigue

- Being obsessed with how much you can eat or what you can eat

- Persistent dizziness, headache, or nausea because of low blood sugar

- Hair loss due to lack of essential nutrients

- Constipation due to lack of fiber, protein, vitamins, or liquids

- The potential to develop eating disorders

- Sleep disorder

Most people will not experience these side effects at a severe level. They will also disappear after a while. However, for some people, this problem can be painful and durable. If so, you might want to stop intermittent fasting until you are looking for medical advice.

Can Athletes try Intermittent Fasting?

Some athletes vowed intermittent fasting as a way to improve athletic performance. However, there is a mixture of research on this. Some evidence shows that training duration and intensity will suffer if you do not consume enough carbohydrates. At the same time, studies show that intermittent fasting offers benefits for athletes. Some of the potential benefits include:

- Growth hormone increases. This helps to boost your bone growth, muscle, and cartilage.

- It improves immune function.

- It improves your metabolic flexibility so you can adapt more easily between energy sources. Your body will be better able to use carbs or fat as a source of fuel.

- It will also allow you to burn fat for much longer before your body switches to carbs. So, your insulin will stay low, and your post-exercise recovery will improve.

- Intermittent fasting reduces inflammation, aiding post-exercise recovery. When you are training, you incur a large amount of inflammation you must recover from—however, the faster that inflammation subsides, the better. Intermittent fasting can speed the process up.

However, there are some concerns. These include:

- Intermittent fasting can cause troubled testosterone due to the impact of muscle protein synthesis.

- You may find it challenging to eat enough calories to allow to get muscle.

Is it Safe for Women to Fast?

Many experts say that it is very safe for women to fast. However, there is evidence that women have greater sensitivity to hunger signals. When the body feels hunger, it increases the production of ghrelin and leptin, a hunger hormone. This causes negative energy balance and, often, changes in the wild mood as a result. Women are also more susceptible to other hormonal imbalances if they do Intermittent fasting. This can cause difficulties in menstrual cycles. It can also interfere with a stimulation of thyroid hormones and this could be problematic for who suffers from autoimmune conditions. That does not mean that women cannot try fasting intermittently. That just means that they need to care more. It might be better for women to start with a softer form than intermittent fasting. For example, you can start with fast 12 hours instead of 16. Some women improve rapidly with intermittent fasting, while others feel they are not suitable for them. You need to experiment to see if it works for you.

Can Children try Intermittent Fasting?

There is no extraordinary evidence to say whether it is safe for children to try it or not. Some experts say that it's okay, especially for those who are overweight. Others say it's a bad idea because children go through a short growth period. Children need enough calories to support their development and growth. Children need to eat quite a lot of protein, vitamins, and minerals. If they are not enough, they can become sick. It might be wise to talk to the doctor before putting a child on an intermittent fasting diet.

Is Fasting Unhealthy?

It's just natural for people to ask if fasting isn't healthy. Those who praise traditional dietary virtues say that fasting can slow down your metabolism. This can cause you to gain weight, not lose it. Therefore, these people said fasting is not healthy for your body. However, this does not happen at all. People have fasted for centuries without harmful effects. Studies conducted on people during Ramadan have shown that expanded fasting does not cause most people health problems. However, there are some problems to remember. Fasting is not for everyone. Some people find it difficult to adjust it to their lives. They struggled to maintain this lifestyle for a long time. They may find it difficult to socialize, work, and exercise around fasting. This can cause an inconsistent meal schedule that might have unhealthy consequences. But there are several other problems to consider too. Some people try to start losing touch with signals that tell them they are complete and hungry. This can make it challenging to stay on intermittent fasting in the long run without developing eating disorders. Some people who are vulnerable to eating disorders are obsessed with eating. Some binge during their eating window. Others encourage their fasting further and further and become transfixed by not eating. It's essential to approach intermittent fasting carefully if you have an irregular dining history. Overall, intermittent fasting can be perfect for you. This can help you manage weight effectively and avoid obesity. This can increase your metabolism and insulin resistance. It can also reduce inflammation and improve your cell repairs and support a healthier digestive tract.

Who Should Avoid Intermittent Fasting?

There are groups of people who must be careful when they do intermittent fasting. Even though they might not need to avoid this lifestyle altogether, they need to be careful. The first group is children. Children grow and develop. Therefore, they need enough calories every day. They also need to get enough nutrients in the form of minerals and vitamins. Without sufficient protein, they can't grow well, and this can lead to several problems. Diseases such as scurvy can be caused by a lack of vitamins. Even though some experts suggest that children can try intermittent fasting, it must be approached carefully. Patients with diabetes must also be careful when they do intermittent fasting. Intermittent fasting indeed has some potential benefits for diabetics. This is because of the effect on insulin levels and blood sugar. However, there are several possible hazards. If you fast and suffer from diabetes, your blood sugar levels can drop very low. This is especially possible if you take medication to control the condition. When someone doesn't eat, blood sugar levels will be lower. Medication for diabetes could then drop it even further, leading to hypoglycaemia. Those with diabetes may feel faint, experience severe tremors, or even have a coma in this condition. Another problem is leading to your blood sugar level that can be too high when you eat. This can happen if you consume many carbohydrates. If you have diabetes, always talk to a health professional before starting an intermittent fasting. You also need to be aware of symptoms of low blood sugar levels. As long as you are careful about what you eat and avoid hard workouts, you won't have any problems whatsoever. The third groups that may want to avoid intermittent fasting are pregnant and lactating women. The doctors usually recommend that these groups not try intermittent fasting. This is because nutrition is essential in these stages of a woman's life - not only does she need to feed herself, but also her baby. Therefore, she needs to consume enough calories and nutrients to sustain two people. This can be difficult when you fast on an intermittent basis. Because it should only be tried under medical supervision.

That being said, there are no severe contraindications for a post-menopausal woman to start learning about the benefits of an intermittent fasting diet! So, what are you waiting for to get started?

What Does Science Say? The Must-Know Effects of Intermittent Fasting on Health and Aging

Intermittent fasting, as we have seen, consists of a window of time in which you fast and another in which you eat. Actually, this practice is not new, as it has been used for centuries. However, without any doubt, in recent years, it has experienced an increase in popularity because it has also been used by big international stars to lose weight and improve the quality of life. One point above all: From 2010 until today, the search in search engines has grown by 10,000%. Stars, from Jennifer Aniston to Fiorello (an Italian showman), have extolled its benefits! Still, even the scientific community agrees: fasting - if done well - is practical and suitable for our bodies.

Most talked about is intermittent fasting, which limits food intake to only the 8-hour window of the day, followed by 16 consecutive hours without food. Among the benefits: rapid weight loss, increased concentration, improved cardiovascular health, and prevention of many diseases such as type 2 diabetes. This happens because you lose visceral fat, which is the most dangerous to your health. Therefore, blood sugar levels and insulin drop dramatically. Some experts claim intermittent fasting reduces inflammatory levels and cholesterol. Anyway, most of the studies have been carried out in mice, which of course, is suitable for. Research conducted in humans has indicated that it is safe - except in some cases, for example, for those who suffer from diabetes - but it is equally effective for losing weight in as many other diets as possible. There is—however, interesting work certifying that the time at which to eat meals can be healthy.

The opinion of science

A review of the recently published literature in the New England Journal of Medicine checking more than 70 studies published on the most common type of intermittent fasting: Method 5: 2 (which provides two days of calorie restrictions per week) and Method 16: 8, Limiting food intake in a limited period during the day, in this case, 8 hours. Among the benefits of this diet appear:

- slowing of aging and age-related diseases (cancer, heart disease, diabetes)

- loss of weight and fat mass

Many studies have shown that reducing caloric intake and intermittent fasting extend the life and reduce the risk of developing various diseases. In 1997, a study conducted by Weindruch and Sohal and published in the New England Journal of Medicine stated that, in laboratory mice, reducing food availability had a positive effect on life expectancy and aging processes. The proposed explanation for this benefit is reduced production of free radicals (responsible for oxidative stress). What the researchers didn't know was that the mice had no sense of delay: given several foods that should be enough for the entire day, they consumed it in a few hours, spending the remaining hours fasting until a next food was delivered. This realization has provided a solution for several in-depth studies of dietary regimens covering fasting and ketogenesis (i.e., energy production from nutritional allowances stored in body tissues) induced by them. Several studies show that intermittent fasting has health benefits.

This not only depends on weight loss and reduces the free radical production: fasting awakens ancestral cellular resources that regulate blood sugar utilization, increase stress resistance, suppress inflammation, and oxidative stress. Nevertheless, most people living in the developed world eat three meals a day, sometimes with snacks in between. How do you set us? A review published in the New England Journal of Medicine summarizes evidence gathered so far in fasting and its effects.

How metabolism changes during intermittent fasting

The primary nutrients in our cells are sugars (primarily glucose) and fatty acids. After eating, the excess fat is stored in adipose tissue in the form of triglycerides; during fasting, to provide the body with fuel it needs for its primary process, this triglyceride is broken down glycerol and fatty acids, which in turn is used as an energy source. The liver changes the fatty acids into a ketone body, which provides energy to many organs (especially the brain). During fasting: the level of the ketone body rises in the blood about 8-12 hours after consuming the last food (unlike, for example, rodents, in which they begin to rise after 4-8 hours). The switch from glucose to fatty acids and the ketone body causes essential changes in the body: the ketone body, in fact, is also a signal molecule, which regulates gene expression and production of substances related to aging. Many studies have indicated that intermittent fasting benefits are not only associated with those related to weight loss: metabolic changes affect the regulation of glucose levels, blood pressure and heart rate, stress resistance, and loss of stomach fat. On this basis, a process called a metabolic switch will occur: usually, after eating, glucose is used to produce energy, while fat is stored in the fatty tissue in the form of triglycerides. However, during the fasting windows, triglycerides are broken down into fatty acids and glycerol, which produce energy. The fatty acids are converted by the liver into the ketone body, an essential energy source during fasting, especially for the brain. When we eat, the food is broken down by specific enzymes found in our intestines and then end up as a molecule in our blood circulation system. Carbohydrates, especially pasta, non-Wholemeal bread, and rice, are quickly broken down into sugar, which our cell used for energy. If this sugar is not used, it is stored in fat cells. Simply put, they become overweight. Insulin is responsible for this work. Between two meals, as long as we are not a snack, the insulin level goes down, and our fat cells can release sugar stored to use it for energy. We lose weight in this situation. The entire intermittent diet theory is based on insulin levels which are pretty low enough to lose weight. During intermittent fasting, therefore, the body alternates its energy sources, glucose, and the ketones. This alternation in the use of energy fuel stimulates an adaptive cellular response that can increase the regulations of blood glucose levels, reduce inflammation, and increase protection from oxidative stress (related to diseases associated with aging.

Be warned, however: according to studies, intermittent fasting is not suitable for everyone; in fact, it would be best avoided for:

- Those who suffer from eating disorders and nervous hunger.

- Pregnant or lactating women.

- Those who suffer from thyroid disorders.

- Those who suffer from diabetes type 1 or type 2.

However, I always remember that before starting this path, it is essential to consult a doctor or nutritionist.

Stress resistance

Unlike what we do today, our ancestors did not eat 3-5 times a day but ate when the opportunity arose. Over time, their bodies adapted to develop creativity and physical strength even in fasting situations, allowing them to find food in any food. Currently, many studies show that most organisms respond to fasting with specific mechanisms that will enable them to tolerate and overcome difficulties and restore balance. In practice, cells answer to fasting by setting up a stress adaptation response: in fact, they increase antioxidant defence, reduce inflammation, and implement DNA repair mechanisms. In animals and humans that have repeatedly experienced fasting, this adaptive mechanism is durable, increasing resilience and resistance to diseases.

The effects on health and aging

After about a century of learning, it was concluded that restrictions on calories (i.e., reduce food intake) extend life. At present, it seems that this consequence is not only related to a quantitative food deficit, but also for the fasting regimen. However, this effect is influenced by various factors, such as species, gender, age, diet, and genetic factors. In addition to increasing life expectancy, it appears that intermittent fasting also increases several aspects of health.

In some studies, people who experience intermittent fasting have shown about other subjects who only reduce caloric intake, not only the same rate of weight loss but also a more significant reduction in thickness around the abdomen and better insulin sensitivity. Not only that, physical and cognitive performance (muscle endurance and intellectual capacity) also seem to increase when food intake decreases.

Practical applications

On Japanese Okinawa Island, a traditional diet includes intermittent fasting. Their diet is based on low-calorie elements but rich in nutrients (such as potatoes, legumes, beans, vegetables); This population is known to have a deficient level of diabetes mellitus and obesity and an extremely long life. These benefits also seem consistent in clinical studies of short-term intermittent fasting. At the same time, data is more controversial in long-term studies. From a cardiovascular health perspective, it has been observed that intermittent fasting increases many indicators of welfare, such as blood pressure levels, resting heart rate, and blood triglyceride levels, cholesterol, and it reduces oxidative stress related to development of atherosclerosis. It appears that overeating, especially during adulthood, predisposes to development of stroke, dementia, and Parkinson's disease. In animal studies, intermittent fasting seems to delay onset of these diseases. Still, there are no reliable clinical studies on humans.

What about cancer? According to recent studies, conducted on the animals, calorie restrictions and the fasting day of alternative days have been shown to reduce the risk of developing many cancers. This effect seems to be related to changes in cancer cell metabolism. In humans, the story is different. Many clinical trials are ongoing or almost complete: the initial results seem to show the benefits of fasting regimen, but we must wait for conclusive data to have reliable evidence.

Aside from the various health benefits related to intermittent fasting, combining this practice into daily life is not easy:

1. Breaking the habit of eating three times a day and countless snacks is not easy, and advertising and marketing spread everywhere do not help in this regard.

2. Starting intermittent fasting is not easy: most people experience anger, irritability, and difficulty concentrating; this usually disappears in a month.
3. Even among physicians, there is a lack of habit of prescribing intermittent fasting regimens: assistance nutritionists or nutritionists are very important to ensure a balanced macro and micro nutritional intake while changing the amount and time of food.

Why the Right Mindset is More Important Than Diet

Mindset, how could we translate this word? We could translate it as "mentality," but it would be better to call it a "mental approach". If I start this chapter from mindset, changing the right mental approach is crucial if we want to lose weight without suffering diets if we're going to understand more how our body works and diet more consciously to feel good. Your mindset is the most important aspect to manage and cultivate when you want to reach your fitness goal. It's infinitely more important than the diet you're on! Most diets don't work because controlling food by following strict rules creates more discomfort than long-term positive effects: yes, we'll probably lose weight, but it's also true that we'll be forced to control everything we do, we'll feel guilty about craving the food we can't have, we'll feel doomed to follow an eating plan that leaves us little choice, depriving us of the joys of food. Sooner or later, the body rebels against this deprivation. But there is a way out. Start with our mindset, that is, change our mental approach to our lifestyle and nutrition. First of all, I want to tell you something: it works. You lose weight more slowly, but you lose weight without dieting.

First of all, what is mindset? We can describe the mindset as a set of ideas, beliefs, and attitudes with which we relate to the world. Obviously, our mindset dramatically influences our daily actions and habits, how we "deal" with the world and interact with others. Why is the set of our daily thoughts and actions more important than this or that diet that we are trying or that we have already failed?

It has been statistically reported that most people who go on a standard diet end the journey after a year with several pounds more than where they started. The most important thing when starting a diet is to understand that only by developing a mindset that allows you to change your habits, in the long run, will you be able to succeed in pursuing and maintaining your goals. Change your relationship with food, deal with stress through meditation, and enjoy tranquillity, sleep quality has never been the primary goal of a diet program, or at least not the most commercial.

This is why the idea of developing the correct mindset to create new eating habits is quite innovative when the first structured diet coaching path is introduced. And do you know why coaching in nutritional work? Because it doesn't only work in the short term and allows you to get the weight you want by changing mindset, exploring the relationship with food, changing lifestyle, and the eating behaviour. The most important thing is to understand that only by developing your willingness and discipline will you succeed in chasing and maintaining your goals. The road to losing weight, or in terms of any external transformation path, cannot be separated from inner work: you need to change, of course, from the inside out.

Why doesn't the classic dietary approach work?

Calories and weight are the main focus of most known diets on the market. Usually, when starting a diet regimen, one must obey restrictions and follow weight claims to measure success or failure. Unfortunately, this approach encourages an unhealthy relationship with food and evaluating with an increase in stable obesity rates, does not work. In the long run, controlling food with strict rules creates more interference than benefits in results, fitness, and self-esteem. Another problem that this approach ignores is that weight loss is not solely about eating "what" needs to be eaten. You may know this yourself: the eating decision you make each day is greatly influenced by the emotions you feel, the time you have, the stress you have built up, and the expectations you have. Therefore, it is necessary to look at all these aspects in a right way. The best thing you can do to achieve rapid progress is to implement a path with a diet coach - many people improve their mealtime behaviour after several meetings. However, you can still adopt some strategies on your own.

Why is it important to develop the right mindset, and how do I get started? There is a way out, and it works: start working on your mindset, change your mental approach to change your lifestyle and diet. But let's get more specific. Even in nutrients, you need a confident attitude, which is a consistent way of achieving a long-awaited goal. It is impossible to think of achieving results without effort. Still, if we have the plan to succeed, we will understand the lower level of effort. The motivation to play sports and the motivation to take a diet comes from the desire to see yourself differently and achieve specific goals. The question is, how much do you care about that goal and how much about nothing in the life you always have? Depending on your priorities, you will see the diet as a means to achieve the goal, unlike others who, regardless of who they go to, will have the excitement for two weeks and then abandon the diet, whatever it is. You, like everyone else, definitely have an idea of what it means to eat healthily: eat more vegetables and fewer food calories, pay attention to the quality of food you put onto the table, get more sports, and so on. Of course, if you make effort every day to improve these aspects, being overweight will disappear. And here we get to the second point, the choice is free: every day you are called to make many choices and many of them concern food. The problem arises because when you are on a diet, or you have to follow a particular food plan, you finally feel locked up, and you don't feel free because the regime seems imposed on you.

Well, we all have a rough idea of what it means to eat healthy. This idea is not the same for everyone, but we can say that it is based on some common notions.

- Eat less if we tend to overeat and reduce alcohol
- Eat more fruits and vegetables and less calorie dense foods
- Pay attention to the quality of the food we put on the table: where does it come from? How nutritious is it? Is it industrially processed, and how much? Does it have unnecessary ingredients, so would I be able to make a healthier version at home?
- Getting more exercise

If we will pay attention to even 1 of these things every day and try to implement our lives, we will get healthy, and overweight will disappear. Next, they are valuable things for us, and here we come to second point: free choice. Every day we are called to make many choices. Many of them regard nutrients. When we are on a diet or follow the food plan, we finally feel locked up, not free, because the food plan seems to enact us. Whether we do this or we don't lose weight. Whether we do this or gain weight. If we don't do this, we will never be better. If we don't do this, we will lose control. Well: in fact, no one forces us to do something we don't want, even not a doctor. The choice is ours; that's the thing we have to say to ourselves at any time.

I can choose to eat, but then I know the consequences. I will feel guilty, feel sick, have flatulence, etc. I can choose to eat a small piece of pizza, or share one with friends, or freeze half: this way I can manage, for example, to eat pizza twice a week, but in a more balanced way, accompanied with vegetables. You are the ruler of your choice; you are the person who decides freely, consciousness, to have behaviour or another one. Suppose you realize this, and no one forces you. Still, you are a person who consciously manages life (you don't need a boss, a teacher, guide), you automatically change your mindset. In that case, you change your mental approach, and you get rid of the idea that you need control outside you to be able to lose weight.

I know it might look complicated, but with a bit of effort, we can tell ourselves every day that we are people who choose how to behave on the table and improve ourselves according to the four directions of nutrition and healthy living for all. In this way, we will lose weight not depending on the diet, not on the plan, but on us. Be aware that the final choice is always yours: You can choose to "throw yourself" on the food and remove all the progress made on the first sign of failure, but you know what the consequences are in guilt and discomfort. The concept of self-responsibilities that I have just introduced wants to emphasize that you are always the ultimate decision-maker: You decide freely, in consciousness, to adopt behaviour than others. If you are aware of this, you can change your mindset and get rid of the idea that you need this or a diet to lose weight. With this, I am not saying that having a road map or eating regimen must be wrong: the important thing is to also grow the right mental approach that is strategically related to the goals and techniques. I know it might look complex, but with a bit of effort, you can start every day to tell yourself that you choose how to behave: this way, losing weight will no longer depend on a particular diet or plan, but on you.

Mindset is critical in dieting to lose weight. Start training your willpower muscle by practicing self-control in simple things, like checking your snack portion and not reacting if someone teases you or trying not to check your Facebook timeline every three minutes. And finally, celebrate your success, even a small one. Any ideas? Try a new meditation, pamper yourself with a massage or beauty treatment, treat yourself to a new piece of clothing to show off with pride! In everything, to succeed, you need the right mindset. Some tips to get you started on a structured diet path:

- Write down what you consume during the day.

- How much to eat (quantity).

- The amount of alcohol you drink for a day, week, and month.

If I told you how many people don't reach a goal because of the amount of alcohol they consume, you might be speechless... As with the nutrition, for example, some concepts are established: if we want to improve aesthetics, we must remember that alcohol must be drastically reduced, if not eliminated. Some people have an excellent aesthetic despite drinking alcohol every day. They are a unique case and obviously do not represent the rule. So, as said many times before: want to lose weight? You need to eat less! You want to gain weight? You need to eat more. These rules are as trivial and superficial as it gets. So now let's see the mindset in nutrition.

The 3 rules for those who follow a diet:

RULE 1: MAKE A PLAN

You need to write a food journal of what you eat. Set goals to change two habits in your routine. Let's use an example to be clearer. Let's pretend that your goal is to lose weight. Do you use to drink alcohol every day and consume pasta for lunch and dinner? Very well. Let's leave everything unchanged except for these 2 aspects. There are no changes to breakfast or lunch and dinner except these two details: one day we will not drink alcohol, but we will consume good pasta at lunch and dinner, while the second day we can drink half a glass of wine, but we can consume pasta only at lunch or only at dinner. The quantity is the same we will obviously consume in just one meal, that is it is not possible to make up for what we will eat in two days!

RULE 2: VALUATE EVERY SMALL OR LARGE GOAL YOU REACH

Whenever we achieve a goal, big or small, think about valuing it. There is no point in focusing on what we expected. Big dreams come from achieving more modest goals.

RULE 3: HAVE A FOCUS

The third rule is the one we will focus on. The focus is knowing exactly the purpose you are fighting for and being motivated to achieve it. Goal must be clearly achieved and not in jest. Unfortunately, many people want to get in shape. Still, they delegate the responsibility because they don't achieve that goal to a third party. This is the most natural reaction. But failure is often driven by a lack of methods and continuity in the process. Time is the necessary requirement. If you have fitness you don't like, and maybe you keep making the same mistakes for years, thinking about building a particular physical type halfway through is pure utopia! Keep in mind that you can ask an expert in the field; the foundation of it all is centred around you. A healthy diet and exercise are a must-have combination.

People who will diet without working out will not shape their bodies the way they want to. Those who will only devote two or three hours a week to working out should know that it will be challenging to get the shape they want without a structured diet. Since being overweight puts you at risk for many health problems, you may need to set up a weight loss plan to avoid these risks and prevent disease. But what should your long-term goal be? What short-term goals should you set to help you get there? You have a better chance of reaching your goals if you make sure the weight loss plan you use is reasonable and sensible, to begin with.

Here are some guidelines from experts in choosing plans and weight loss goals.

1. Be realistic

Long-term weight loss plans are highly ambitious. For example, if you weigh 180 pounds and your plan is to consider 120 - even if you haven't weighed 120 since you were 16 and are now 45 - that's not a realistic weight loss target. The body mass index or BMI is a good indicator of whether you need to shed pounds. According to the National Institutes of Health, the perfect BMI range is between 19 and 24.9. If your BMI exceeds this target and is between 25 and 29.9, you are considered overweight. If your BMI exceeds even this range, you are considered obese - any number above 30 is in the obesity range. From this point of view, you will need a reasonable weight-loss plan that agrees with the required BMI based on your height because this is the main factor that will affect your BMI.

2. Set appropriate objectives

Using a weight loss plan for psychological vanity is less helpful than losing weight to improve your health. You have taken a big step forward if you decide to undergo a weight loss plan that includes proper exercises and meals, so you'll feel better and have more energy to do something positive with your life.

3. Focus on doing, not losing

Instead of thinking that you will lose little weight this week, you will exercise this week. This will definitely be a reasonable weight-loss plan. Keep in mind that your weight cannot be kept entirely under control in just one week, but your behavior and habits can.

4. Build bit by bit

Your short-term weight loss plan should not be "pie-in-the-sky". This means that when you've never exercised, you can't start out thinking you can run a marathon. Your best plan for this week should be to find the best steps to walk the first leg of your weight loss journey and start your training.

5. Keep up the self-encouragement

All-O's attitude - nothing makes you fail. Learn to evaluate your efforts objectively and fairly. If you miss any goals, look ahead to next week. It is not necessary to be perfect. However, self-encouragement must be part of your weight loss plan. Otherwise, you will ultimately just fail.

6. Use measurable measures

Saying that you will be more positive this week or that you will be really serious this week is not a goal you can measure and should not be part of your weight loss plan. This is another reason why you should incorporate exercises into your weight loss plan and focus on them. You need to be able to calculate consecutive treaties to be successful in your project. The point is that people need to make a weight loss plan that will remain so, just a plan. You have to act by combining goals that will motivate you to success.

So, if you're someone with a bit of a mindset in nutrition, start by assessing what your end goal is and try to remember it when you want to drink too much beer or find a reason not to go to the gym. Three simple words to repeat to yourself day after day: consistency, continuity, perseverance.

This is the action we take that makes up the material we make up our idea of ourselves. We then create a definition of what characteristics of our personality!

Which Type of Intermittent Fasting Should You Choose According to Your Body

There are different types of intermittent fasting. Usually, the difference will depend on the person and how they adapt the method to suit their needs. However, the basics of the lunch window and the fasting window will always be essential. Remember that it doesn't matter which method you choose. All the different techniques will reap the expected results. You must select a plan that is comfortable for you. When the way you choose is easy for you to follow, the chances of following it will be much higher.

Initially, suppose you are new to intermittent fasting. In that case, you will want to slow down and have a longer meal window and a shorter fasting window. It will take anywhere from 15 days to a month for your body to adjust to the new mode of nutrition. There is no doubt that you will most likely face resistance and cravings from your body. This is normal. However, most people are used to eating all the time they are awake. Limiting mealtimes can be stressful at first. Rest assured that your body will adapt over time, and you will be surprised to see your appetite gradually decrease. You will also feel more alert, vital, active, energetic, and slimmer as you go on. Now let's look at some of the intermittent fasting methods.

- Intermittent Fasting Method 1

The first method is the most popular of all. It is very effective and relatively easy to follow. The rule is that men need to fast for 16 hours and women for 14 hours. They will have a meal window of 8 hours and 10 hours, respectively. So, it is essential to maintain consistency in this mode. Otherwise, your body will get confused and will inhibit the results. It is recommended that you plan your meals around your workout. For example, if your meal window ends at 7:00 pm, you should train around 5:30 pm and consume your food before 7:00 pm. Or you can start your meal window after your workout. This way, the body will have nourishment to improve muscles, etc.

- Intermittent Fasting Method 2

The second method is much stricter. The rule says that you have to fast for 20 hours a day and eat only 1 great food every night. This is supposed to be what our ancestors did. Many people who adopt this method to date have seen significant benefits to their health. Initially, you might not want to use the following procedure: called ORI. It would be a better idea to start with the ORI method and gradually reduce your meal window over time until you get to fast for 20 hours without discomfort. You should know that the ORI method allows some small foods during fasting window. However, there are rules about what you can and cannot eat. So, you have to watch your diet and stay on the list of approved foods. This is definitely one of the strictest methods.

- Intermittent Fasting Method 3

The third method of intermittent fasting is known as stop eating. The rules of this fast are pretty simple. You will fast for 24 hours two or three times a week. On the days you don't fast, you can eat what you want without worrying about that. This way, your overall calorie consumption for this week will be deficient, and you will lose weight. Since you are allowed to eat whatever, you want during the meal window, you will not lose your favorite foods. This can provide relief to many people who are afraid to give up the food they love. However, 24 hours off from eating can be very difficult for many people.

How do you decide?

The truth is, you need to analyze your eating habits, your sleeping patterns, your work requirements, etc. You need to adjust the fasting that suits you. If you work at night, you can't get fast all night because you will be hungry. So, you need to fit your sleeping hours into your fasting window and maybe start your meal window 6 hours after you wake up.

Of course, this assumes that you adopt the first type of intermittent fasting. If you have social activities, it can be challenging to follow an intermittent fasting program. Sooner or later, your fasting will damage your social life.

Again, you have to manage it. Even the actor, Hugh Jackman, was on the intermittent fasting program while practicing for the Wolverine movie and had to make sure he was attached to the meal window despite his busy schedule. In the end, you have to choose the method that you think will work for you. Don't be too ambitious or overdo it by choosing right away with a 24-hour fast on the first day.

This will most likely be torture. Eventually, you may give up and eat. Then, you may experience feelings of guilt and feel like you have failed. This is where most people have thrown in the towel. They think they have failed when in reality, they have only set unreasonable goals. The key to success is to make progress measurable with reasonable goals.

"Inch by inch, life's a cinch. Yard by yard, life is hard."

A Day in the Life of IF

It will be challenging to assign the same plan for everyone, as each individual has different needs and schedules. However, here are some tips you must know when planning your program. Before you know the goals to follow to adopt an intermittent fasting plan to lose weight, you need to see the number of daily calories to ingest. You need to know how many calories to eat to be in a calorie deficit of about 500 calories every day. On the other hand, if you are trying to structure a muscular body, you need to go into a caloric surplus, thus consuming all the calories in the meal window. This could be really difficult if you consume a lot of calories.

However, you will be less likely to gain weight. If you are happy with your weight, you can continue eating what you are eating now. It will be a good idea to check if your diet is healthy. All you need to do is adjust all the foods in your meal window.

Know your schedule
Intermittent fasting generally doesn't focus on the food you eat. It focuses on time. The time of your meals and cutting time is a track of intermittent fasting. Therefore, it is necessary to adhere to indicative windows. Many people who begin intermittent fasting usually find that their lives are controlled by their food windows and fasting windows. They need to constantly check the time and plan things. All of these inconveniences can be avoided with proper planning. Look at your schedule and your preferences. What time do you wake up? What time is your lunch break at work? Do you prefer to eat after you wake up, or do you choose to sleep on a full stomach? You must know your schedule and preferences. If you like to sleep with a full stomach, you may need to schedule your meal window to start 6 hours after waking up. What if you work and are hungry? Can you rest up to eat your first meal when your meal window is open? All of this is a consideration you need to remember when planning your fast.

How much food will you eat?

Some people may prefer to eat during the meal window with a few snacks. Others may choose for 1 or 2 large meals. Either way, it's not a problem ... but it is necessary to know what you like and plan for it.

When have you been exercising?

Your ideal is to start a regular sports program. However, you need to know what time you are going to exercise. Will you exercise on an empty stomach? It is essential to eat after exercise to get the fuel it needs, which will also increase your metabolic rate. So, plan your meal window so that you can eat after your workout.

How to Maximize Your Intermittent Fasting Results

Are you ready to try intermittent fasting? Are you doing it to lose weight or for other benefits? You may want to maximize the results. Fortunately, you can do a few things to get as much help from your eating regimen as possible. Here we look at some things you can try to accelerate your weight loss and get back to the body you had a few years ago. To maximize the yield of intermittent fasting, you have to choose the proper regimen.

As you can see, there are different types of intermittent fasting diets. Not all of them are suitable for everyone. You need to find the one that works well for your lifestyle and makes your life easier. Consider that when you choose the proper regimen, you'll stick with it for the long term. So, here are some questions to ask yourself to help you choose wisely. Have you been eating healthy? Fasting is more difficult if you're eating a standard American diet. That's because a junk food diet is high in carbs, full of sugar, and very addictive. If you jump straight to extreme fasting, you will experience sugar withdrawal symptoms. This makes it challenging to maintain your new diet.

If you usually eat processed food regularly, try starting with a short fasting window. In the meantime, detox from sugar and start eating cleaner. Stop snacking and introduce whole foods into your diet. You can then increase the fasting window if necessary. On the other hand, if you eat healthy food, you can start with a longer fasting window. Can you manage to go a long time without eating? Some people can manage fasting for the entire day. Other people can only manage a few hours. You may need to experiment. Focus on how fasting makes you feel. If you struggle for a long time, choose methods like 5:2 or 16:8. If you feel comfortable, you may slowly lengthen your fasting window.

How to set yourself up. It is easier to fast if you are busy and disturbed by thoughts of food. If you fast at work or when you are working on something, you may feel less hungry. If you exercise, you may want to end your fasting window after exercising. If you answer these questions, you will be put in the best place to choose the proper regimen to suit your life and preferences. This will give you the best chance for success.

Adding in Keto

Some experts say that if you combine intermittent fasting with a keto diet, you will lose more weight. So, what's the point? The keto diet is a unique method of eating in which most of the calories come from healthy fats. The remaining calories come from protein. Carbohydrates are drastically reduced, if not excluded, from this type of diet. Consuming a high content of health-beneficial fats prompts your body to burn fat, not sugar, to produce energy. If you reduce your daily carbohydrate intake, your body will use fat reserves to perform daily activities. This mechanism produces ketones that are then used as fuel for energy. This process is known as ketosis. Hence the name "Keto." Like intermittent fasting, the keto diet has several benefits: it can speed up the weight loss process, reduce blood sugar levels and improve brain function. Many people say that the ketogenic diet helps reduce problems such as diabetes and obesity. If you combine the keto diet with intermittent fasting, the amount of time you are in ketosis increases. This will offer several long-term benefits on your body: you'll regain the energy you had when you were 30, you'll feel a reduced sense of hunger, and all of this will have an anti-aging effect on your body and mind, speeding up so hungry and accelerating your weight loss.

Common Intermittent Fasting Mistakes to Avoid

There are several mistakes made by people when it comes to intermittent fasting. All of these mistakes can be avoided.

Mistake 1 – Giving up too fast

You have to understand that intermittent fasting is the opposite of what most people are used to. Adopting the Intermittent fasting method will not be accessible at first. Don't give up just because you may make some small mistakes. It is almost inevitable that you will make mistakes or give in to temptation. You may get hungry and eat something, only to feel guilty and curse yourself for being weak. You might decide that the whole plan has failed and stop. This is a process that is established through habit and glorified by many beginners. Never stop! If you do give in and eat a snack, stick with less caloric foods. Over time, your appetite will diminish, and you will be more disciplined. It will be easier to stick with that plan. In fact, usually after two or three weeks, most people on intermittent fasting find it harder to consume all their calories in the meal window. They now feel like they have too much to eat and too little time to eat their meals from excessive food cravings. You will be amazed to see how quickly your body is adjusting. Resist, and you will prevail.

Mistake 2 – Poor planning

As mentioned before, time is significant in the intermittent fasting program. If you plan poorly, you will constantly be watching the clock. Intermittent fasting can be stressful at first, but it is just a matter of habit. You should not be stressed because of poor planning.

Mistake 3 – Being too ambitious

There are different types of intermittent fasting. Many beginners want quick weight loss results. They adopt the fasting diet, which involves 24-hour fasting or drastic calorie-cutting combined with intermittent fasting. Slow and steady wins the race. If you try to do too much too fast, the whole process will become torture and stressful. It will only be a matter of time when your willpower fails you, and you stop. So, start small and make a shorter fasting window. As the days progress, you can gradually increase the length of your fasting window.

Mistake 4 – Not watching their diet

All calories are not made equal. Getting 400 calories from one piece of lean meat is different than getting 400 calories from 2 candy bars. Intermittent fasting allows for some concessions with your diet. Still, if you want faster results by losing your fat, you also need to eat a healthy, proper diet. Your diet and intermittent fasting are not mutually exclusive. Combine a healthy eating style with intermittent fasting, and you will burn local fat faster.

Mistake 5 – Not exercising

Yes ... it's hard work. Yes, you can lose weight with intermittent fasting and a healthy diet. However, if you want to be stronger and fitter, you need to exercise. Ideally, you need to have a mixture of cardio and resistance training in your practice. You can keep things interesting by trying different exercises or even other types of exercises. Pilates one day, kickboxing the next, or maybe swimming a few laps on the weekend. The key is to move more and challenge yourself. Exercise is a habit. It is a hard habit to instill, but it is straightforward to lose.

Intermittent fasting will help you lose weight, and exercise will not only speed up the process, but in the long run, it will eliminate excess fat. It is a fact that most people can lose weight but often fail to eliminate excess fat.

The key to training is to build strength and endurance in stages. There are workout days and rest days. Never miss workout days just because you don't feel like it. After doing this, you will find that you have no enthusiasm to train the next day, and before you know it, you have stopped training for three weeks. Now, you need to struggle again to get back into a rhythm. If you don't want to lose momentum, don't stop for too long. One day off is more than enough.

Usually, one day off every three days is enough to give your body a rest. After knowing what a common mistake is, you can avoid it and achieve success with intermittent fasting.

Nutrition Basics: What are Macronutrients and Micronutrients

Nutrition is the basis of human metabolism. Each food plays a specific role in the body, aiding in growth, recovery, and defense against disease. Foods are divided into two categories: macronutrients and micronutrients.

The first group includes carbohydrates, proteins, fats, water, and alcohol (they are essential nutrients for optimal health). The second group contains vitamins and minerals. Macronutrients promote body growth and micronutrients contribute to optimal cell function. Although it is possible to get nutrients through food, dietary supplements may also be necessary, especially for those who lead very active lives or follow low fruit and vegetable intake.

What is a macronutrient? Macronutrients are the building blocks of our bodies and consist of three categories: fats, proteins, and carbohydrates. Some experts include in the list of macronutrients water and alcohol. Still, in the case of water, there is no caloric value. In the case of alcohol instead, it is possible to find a high caloric index; there is no usability for metabolic purposes because this element has no nutritional value. Moreover, alcohol is considered a dangerous substance outside the minimum threshold. All macronutrients provide energy (in the form of calories) and participate in the organism's development, help in defense and reconstruction of the damaged part of the organism.

Types and functions of macronutrients
We mentioned three main types of macronutrients that are important to our diet: carbohydrates, proteins, and fats. All contribute to the well-being of the body and the nutritional needs of our body. Let's see in detail. Carbohydrates are the mainstay of our diet, as they provide energy through calories and are very important for our body.

Carbohydrates take care of three fundamental processes:

-    They trigger vital mechanisms to help the body during daily movement activities and during exercise

-    They allow the central nervous system to function effectively

-    They protect the muscles during intense activity

1 gram of carbohydrates produces 4 calories. The recommended daily intake of carbohydrates is between 45% and 60% of the calories needed each day. We need to know that our body is a huge energy saver, so an excess of carbohydrates leads to weight gain in terms of the fat mass. What should be avoided is food with processed sugar, such as candy or carbonated soft drinks, and excessively processed, such as snacks, chips, etc.

Fats

Fats play a central role in our bodies, providing long-term energy. In addition to this primary function, their reputation as nutrition is often underestimated and hated because of their high-calorie content. 1 gram of fat produces 9 calories, so we must carefully balance their intake in our diet. FATS perform a vital process:

-    They act as energy reserves (even long-term)

-    They protect vital organs

-    They protect the body from cold

-    They transport soluble vitamins

The World Health Organization recommends a daily percentage of calories from fat of less than 30%.

Source of fat

Unsaturated fats are considered the healthiest because they contain many Omega 3 and Omega 6 fatty acids. Our bodies cannot produce these nutrients, so it is necessary to introduce them through food. Fish, especially tuna and mackerel, are known to be the most abundant sources of fatty acids. Still, some vegetables can offer important contributions, such as avocados, grains and flaxseed oil, nuts, cereals, beans, lentils, and peas.

Protein

The structural foundation of our bodies, proteins are essential to living. Without them, we would not exist. Proteins are made up of amino acids, some essential and some non-essential. The former we take in through food, including supplements, while the others are produced by other proteins we take in. There are several functions performed by proteins in our bodies:

-   They create network structures (muscles, hair, organs, etc.).

-   They create structures for substances such as hormones and antibodies

-   They form enzymes that regulate metabolism

-   Participate in body's growth, maintenance, and recovery (protein requirements vary based on activity or age)

Like carbohydrates, 1 gram of protein produces 4 calories. The proper diet covers 10% to 35% of calories from protein each day. We understand that meat and fish are the primary sources of protein. Still, even among vegetables, some foods contribute significantly: nuts, beans, and seeds. A trendy alternative among vegans is Spirulina, an alga with the high protein content, whose supplements can be found in organic supermarkets.

What are micronutrients?

Micronutrients consist of vitamins and minerals. Their purpose is to activate specific chemical reactions in the body, regulate hormonal functions, and prevent disease.

Micronutrients do not provide energy through the calories; however, they are essential for the development of our bodies. Vitamins are organic compounds, while minerals are inorganic compounds, and both are taken in through food. In case of deficiencies due to limited food consumption, both minerals and vitamins can be introduced into the body through supplements.

Type and function of micronutrients

Among vitamins/minerals, twenty-six substances activate several endless chemical reactions, which are essential for the health of our body.

Unlike macronutrients, micronutrients are needed in small quantities. Also, vitamins are divided into two categories: water-soluble (water-soluble) and fat-dissolvable (fat-soluble).

Water soluble vitamins

This type of vitamin is dissolved in water in the body; therefore, we lose significant amounts of soluble vitamins through evacuation, causing vitamin deficiencies.

A solution to this problem is the use of some vitamin supplements. Let's see in detail which is a water-soluble vitamin and where it works:

- Vitamin B2 (riboflavin): Involved in energy production, lipid metabolism, and cellular function.

- Vitamin B3 (Niacin): Produces energy from food.

- Vitamin B5 (Pantothenic Acid): Contributes to the synthesis of fatty acids.

- Vitamin B6 (Pyridoxine): Produces red blood cells and uses sugar reserves for energy.

- Vitamin B7 (Biotin): Helps break down acidic fat, amino acids, and glucose to produce energy.

- Vitamin B9 (folate): Participates in cell division.

- Vitamin B12 (cobalamin): It is essential for the formation of red blood cells and for the functioning of the brain and nervous system; For this reason, it must be supplemented in a vegan and vegetarian diet if low in B12.

- Vitamin C (ascorbic acid): Plays a crucial role in the health of the body by strengthening the immune system.

Fat-soluble vitamins

Fat-soluble vitamins are unlike water-soluble vitamins. Therefore, they are insoluble in water but are absorbed when consumed with foods rich in fat.

- Vitamin A: Important for organic functions.

- Vitamin D: Important for calcium absorption, bone growth, and immune function.

- Vitamin E: Protects cells from damage and contributes to immune function.

- Vitamin K: Important for blood clotting and bone development.

Macrominerals

They represent most of the minerals we need to perform our bodily functions. There are seven in total:

- Calcium: Useful for bone and tooth development; It also assists the muscle function and blood vessel contractions.

- Chloride: Promote fluid balance and interference in production of gastric juice.

- Magnesium: Contribute to blood pressure regulation.

- Phosphorus: Support bone structure and cell membranes.

- Potassium: Electrolyte functions involved in nerve transmission and muscle function.

- Sodium: Electrolytes that function to maintain constant blood pressure and fluid balance.

- Sulfur: part of all vital networks.

Our business agency requires trace minerals in the macromineral amount, which we can see in detail below:

- Iron: provides oxygen to muscle and promotes hormone production.

- Manganese: participate in the metabolism of carbohydrates, proteins, and fats.

- Copper: necessary for the formation of the Tie network and for the control of brain function and nervous systems.

- Zinc: is essential for average body growth, regulating immune function and healing wounds.

- Iodine: management of thyroid function.

- Fluoride: Useful for the development of teeth and bones.

- Selenium: Acts to defend cells and contributed to the excellent health of the thyroid.

The Best Nutrients and Vitamins after 50

Proper nutrition can counteract the aging process in many ways. First, food helps prevent disease. Second, the appropriate nutrition supports the body's health and overall function, allowing its ability to stay strong, vital, in good condition regardless of age. The proper meal is the key to staying healthy, and at age 50, nutrients require a change from what you may have needed in previous years. Essential vitamins and minerals are necessary for skin health to protect against top killers of women such as heart disease, cancer, strokes, and even manage menopausal symptoms.

Never underestimate the voice of nutrition in decelerating the aging process and living a long and healthy life.

Calcium

Calcium is essential for strong bones, and it helps prevent osteoporosis. Also, calcium makes teeth strong, helps the body with blood clotting function, and helps maintain a regular heartbeat. Calcium-rich foods are:

- Milk
- Yogurt
- Okra
- Collard greens
- Soybeans
- White beans
- Spinach
- Kale
- Sardines, salmon, trout, perch

Calcium-fortified foods including oatmeal, cereals, and orange juice.

Vitamin D

Vitamin D helps prevent osteoporosis by supporting calcium absorption, which helps keep bones strong. It also maintains brain and mental health and reduces the risk of depression. It can also control blood pressure and cholesterol levels. This can play an essential role in reducing inflammation and protecting the body from many chronic diseases. Enough vitamin D is easy to absorb if you spend at least 10 to 15 minutes in the sun each day; You can also supplement through diet and vitamin supplements.

Foods rich in vitamin D are:

- Fatty fish, such as tuna, mackerel, and salmon
- Vitamin D fortified foods, such as cereals, dairy products, orange juice, soy milk
- Beef liver
- Cheese
- Egg yolks

Vitamin B1 (Thiamine)

Vitamin B1 or thiamine is needed for brain and nerve cell health and helps the body turn food into energy. CAUTION: Some diuretics and antacids may reduce thiamine levels in body by reducing its absorption, increasing its secretion through urination. Vitamin B1 Food Sources are:

- Liver
- Enriched breads
- Enriched cereals
- Whole grains

Vitamin B3 (Niacin)

Vitamin B3 is necessary for proper digestion and nervous system function. Vitamin B3 supports the skin's ability to retain moisture, helping the body fight off viruses, bacteria, and other antigens.

Niacin also helps the skin eliminate dead cells, allowing newer cells to rise to surface for more radiant, youthful-looking skin. Niacin helps the body turn food into energy. It also helps increase good cholesterol (HDL) while reducing the wrong type (LDL), reducing the risk of heart disease, stroke, and atherosclerosis. Foods rich in niacin are:

- Poultry
- Eggs
- Fish

- Nuts
- Avocados
- Enriched breads

Vitamin B6 (Pyridoxine)

Vitamin B6 helps keep the brain healthy and functioning at its best. This nutrient also plays a vital role in metabolic process and how the body turns food into energy, helping to break down proteins and maintain healthy blood glucose levels. This aids the body in the production of haemoglobin. Foods rich in vitamin B6 are:

- Fish
- Nuts
- Seeds
- Potatoes
- Chickpeas
- Avocados

- Bananas
- Beans
- Oatmeal
- Lean meat
- Poultry

Vitamin B12

Vitamin B12 helps with the production of DNA and red blood cells. It also aids in the metabolic process and helps maintain healthy nerve function. This is important for brain health and the blood function. Recent studies show that vitamin B12 increase concentration levels, treat memory loss, and lift mood and energy levels. One of the main problems regarding vitamin B12 is that 1/3 of people over 50 cannot absorb it from the diet, which can cause neurological and balance problems.

The use of certain medications, often taken by older populations, can cause disruptions in the way B12 is absorbed and metabolized in the body. Foods rich in vitamin B12:

- Fish	- Milk
- Lean meat	- Cheese
- Poultry	- Yogurt
- Eggs	

Folic Acid

Vitamin B9 or Folic acid reduces the risk of anemia, helps keep brain and spinal cord healthy, and produces red blood cells. It also helps in the production of DNA and RNA, creating cell building and new networks. Folic acid helps prevent DNA changes that cause cancer. Research has shown that folate is similar to hormone replacement therapy (HRT), which can help relieve menopause-related hot flashes by disrupting monoamine, serotonin, and norepinephrine.

Foods rich in folic acid are:

- Dark leafy vegetables	- Citrus fruits
- Olive oil	- Broccoli
- Asparagus	- Strawberries
- Brussels sprouts	- Fortified grains
- Beets	- Chickpeas
- Lentils	- Black and kidney beans
- Peanut butter	- Eggs
- Spinach	- Squash
- Melons	- Nuts

Vitamin K

Vitamin K helps the blood clotting process; it helps reduce the risk of heart disease. It is also essential for building and maintaining strong bones. It interferes with blood thinner medications, so be sure to ask your doctor. Foods rich in vitamin K are:

- Eggs
- Cauliflower
- Broccoli
- Asparagus
- Brussels sprouts
- Cabbage

Vitamin C

Vitamin C is an antioxidant that helps remove and prevent damage brought on by free radicals. It also helps heal wounds, helps produce red blood cells, and increases brain chemicals called norepinephrine, making you more focused and alert. Vitamin C also promotes healthy gums and teeth, makes it easier for the body to absorb iron, and helps maintain a healthy immune system. For aging women, the vitamin C helps support eye health. When applied directly to skin, it helps protect it from the harmful effects of the sun. It also gives a more youthful appearance by increasing the collagen production, giving the skin a glow. Foods rich in vitamin C are:

- Broccoli
- Grapefruit
- Kiwi
- Oranges
- Bell peppers
- Potatoes
- Strawberries
- Tomatoes
- Cauliflower
- Citrus fruits

Vitamin A

Aging process makes it increasingly necessary to increase your intake of antioxidants to keep your cells healthy, protect against many diseases, inflammations, and keep your skin healthy and ageless. Vitamin A is essential for bone health. It is also crucial for healthy immunity while applied to the skin shows visible results. When applied topically, facial creams with vitamin A (retinol cream) help reduce signs of sunlight damage, dark under-eye circles, and fine expression lines.

Foods rich in vitamin A are:

- Eggs
- Milk and fortified milk
- Dark leafy vegetables
- Carrots
- Cantaloupe
- Apricots
- Papaya
- Peaches
- Kale
- Guava
- Red peppers
- Pumpkins
- Tomatoes
- Spinach

Vitamin E

Vitamin E is an antioxidant responsible for dissolving essential fat, neutralizing the effects of fat oxidation. It then stops the production of free radicals, which contribute to chronic disease and aging. Vitamin E also promotes a healthy immune system.

The study researches the possibility of its role in preventing degenerative dementia conditions, such as Alzheimer's disease. Research has shown that it helps reduce the risk of atherosclerosis by lowering LDL cholesterol levels. It may also protect the body from the spread of cancer cells by neutralizing the damaging effects of free radicals and may protect against heart disease. Vitamin E is often used in facial creams to moisturize the skin and improve dryness, also used in sunscreen to protect the skin from dangerous UV rays. WARNING: Talk to your doctor if you take blood thinners because vitamin E supplements increase the risk of diluting blood fluid.

Foods rich in vitamin E are:

- Almonds
- Mustard Greens
- Spinach
- Turnip Greens
- Kale
- Swiss chard
- Plant oils
- Olives

- Raw seeds
- Hazelnuts
- Pine Nuts

- Broccoli
- Parsley
- Papaya

Magnesium

More than 300 enzymatic functions require magnesium to function correctly, such as maintaining a healthy heart, strong bones, metabolism, healthy nerve, and muscle function, and regulates blood pressure and blood glucose levels. It also helps absorb calcium in the body. It can help prevent type 2 diabetes. Magnesium helps maintain a healthy heart rhythm. For women, it reduces the risk of high blood pressure.

Foods rich in magnesium are:

- Dark leafy greens
- Fish
- Nuts
- Whole grains

- Beans
- Avocados
- Bananas

Potassium

Potassium is an essential mineral for the optimal functioning of the muscles, heart, kidneys, and nerves. Potassium works with sodium to help maintain the body's water balance. It makes bones strong, helps maintain healthy cellular function, regulates blood pressure levels. This helps reduce the risk of kidney stones, regulates digestion, aids metabolism, increases energy, reduces muscle spasms. In aging, in particular, this mineral can help reduce the risk of heart disease, which is the No. 1 female killer in the United States, and also plays a role in stroke prevention.

Foods rich in potassium are:

- Bananas
- Prunes

- Plums
- Potatoes with skin

- Lentils, Beans
- Sweet potatoes

Zinc

A recent research published in the Journal of Nutritional Biochemistry reports that zinc deficiency can develop with age and can cause weakened immunity and promote inflammation, which is known to trigger aging of the body and chronic diseases, such as type 2 diabetes and cancer and heart disease. Zinc also helps maintain taste and smell. It helps with healing. Some studies show that a combination of antioxidants and zinc can reduce the risk of age-related macular degeneration. Ask your doctor to judge whether you need supplements. Foods rich in Zinc are:

- Scallops
- Pumpkin seeds
- Sesame seeds
- Shrimp
- Lobster

- Crab
- Cooked spinach
- Beans
- Beef
- Wheat germ

Omega-3 Fatty Acids

Omega-3 fatty acids are healthy monounsaturated fats. We can find the marine forms (DHA and EPA) in oily fish. Plant forms contain alpha-linolenic acid or ALA and are found in plant foods, including oils, seeds, and nuts. The first ones, EPA and DHA, can lower high triglyceride levels, reducing the risk of heart disease. Omega-3 fatty acids elevate good HDL cholesterol and lower bad LDL cholesterol. These fats also help reduce risk factors for cancer. Consuming omega-3 fatty acids helps manage mood swings related to menopause and may help prevent depression and depressive symptoms. Omega-3s can also sharpen brain function. The EPA and DHA found in fish oil help relieve joint pain and stiffness in rheumatoid arthritis patients. These nutrients increase the effectiveness of the anti-inflammatory medications. ALA helps reduce body's inflammation and may prevent chronic diseases, including arthritis and heart disease. However, ALA is not as potent as marine sources of omega-3, EPA, and DHA. While no definitive conclusions have been drawn, there is some promising research that omega-3 fatty acids protect against senile dementia and Alzheimer's disease and positively affect gradual age-related memory loss.

Good sources of EPA and DHA are:

- Mackerel
- Wild Caught Salmon
- Anchovies
- Bluefish
- Herring

- Sardines
- Sturgeon
- Lake trout
- Tuna

Good plant sources of ALA are:

- Olives and olive oil
- Walnuts and walnut oil
- Avocados and avocado oil
- Flaxseed and flaxseed oil
- Canola oil
- Soybean oil
- Fortified eggs

- Brussels sprouts
- Kale
- Mint
- Parsley
- Spinach
- Watercress

Iron

Iron is an essential mineral found in the human body's red blood cells, which carry oxygen. Iron deficiency can cause anaemia, where there is a reduction in healthy red blood cells. Iron reduces the risk of certain diseases and promotes healthy immunity.

Foods rich in iron are:

- Red meat
- Beef and chicken liver
- Pork
- Poultry

- Seafood
- Beans
- Dark green leafy vegetables including spinach and kale

- Dried fruit including apricots and raisins
- Iron-fortified bread, pasta and cereals

Fiber

While digestive health and regularity may be the most well-known benefit, the fiber offers additional benefits that are important for good health, especially as they relate to aging. Fiber helps reduce the risk of developing type 2 diabetes, and studies have shown that it lowers blood pressure. Fiber makes you fuller, so you eat less; this helps support healthy weight, which is key to healthy aging and avoiding chronic severe diseases resulting from obesity, such as heart disease, type 2 diabetes, cancer, joint problems. According to research compiled by the Blue Mountains Eye Study by Professor Bamini Gopinath (Westmead Institute for Medical Research Center for Vision Research), there is new evidence that fibers support and promote what is dubbed as "successful aging."

Fiber prevents brain disorders, depression, respiratory problems, cancer, coronary heart disease, and stroke. This study examines more than 1,600 adults aged 50 and older. It focuses on exploring the relationship between carbohydrate intake in aging and a healthy diet. Factors examined include total fiber intake, total carbohydrate intake, glycaemic load and index, and sugar intake. This study found that fiber intake made the most significant difference in "successful aging." The researchers found that the subjects tested who had the highest fiber intake had a nearly 80% greater chance of enjoying a long and healthy life, free of hypertension, type 2 diabetes, depression, dementia, and disability during the 10-year follow-up period.

Foods Rich in Fiber are:

- Vegetables
- Fruits

A Protocol for 16:8 Intermittent Fasting

If you want to start intermittent fasting, you might want to start fasting at 16: 8. This method involves fasting for 16 hours and then having an 8-hour meal window. This is one of the most popular forms of this method. If you are ready to start, here is the protocol for 16: 8 intermittent fasting.

Choosing a meal window

When you are ready to start 16:8 fasting, the first thing you need to do is choose a meal window. These 8 hours can be tailored to fit everyone's needs. Therefore, you can choose the right time to suit your preferences and your lifestyle. Once you have selected the eight hours of your choice, you must limit your food consumption to these hours. How do you choose the right time for you?

Many people prefer meal windows starting from lunch until 8 tonight because they may get more comfortable skipping breakfast and enjoying lunch and dinner at the usual time. They can also add some healthy snacks into their regimen.

For people who prefer to have three meals a day, the window that runs from 9 a.m. to 5 p.m. might be indicated. This allows them to eat breakfast at 9 a.m., have lunch during the day, and then have an early dinner at 4 p.m. Others prefer to wait until the afternoon to break their fast and then for their last meal later in the day before bed. Whatever window you choose, make sure it matches your lifestyle. If you decide it wrong, you won't be able to survive your diet.

Plan healthy food

To maximize the 16: 8 intermittent fasting benefits, you need to eat as healthy as possible. If you feed yourself nutrient-rich food, you will not be hungry or crave unhealthy food. While you may enjoy snacks and treats, you must balance each meal with a variety of foods. Some of the best foods include:

-    Fruits like bananas, oranges, apples, pears, peaches, berries

- Vegetables like tomatoes, leafy greens, cucumbers, broccoli, and cauliflower

- Whole grains like rice, oats, quinoa, buckwheat, and barley

- Healthy fats like olive oil, coconut oil, and avocados

- Lean protein like poultry, fish, seeds, nuts, eggs, and legumes

If you eat Junk Food frequently, you can negate the benefits of this diet. Therefore, you still have to keep an unhealthy choice as possible.

Choose a calorie-free drink

You can have a beverage of your choice during your meal window. If you drink a few bottles of soda, you may not lose any weight! During your fasting window, you must consume only calorie-free drinks. If you consume a beverage containing calories, you are basically harming your eating regimen. Water, green tea, coffee, herbal teas, and sweetener-free tea without milk are good choices. They will also help you control your appetite and keep you hydrated throughout the fasting period.

A Protocol for 24-Hour Intermittent Fasting

If the 16:8 diet is not for you, you might consider the 24-hour fast. This is known as the eat-stop-eat method. This involves one or two non-consecutive days of fasting each week.

Introduction to the Eat-stop-Eat Method

This method was designed by Brad Pilon, who wrote a book on how to eat following this method. The methodology is based on Canadian research on the influences of short-term fasting on metabolic health. The idea behind the Pilon method is to revaluate everything you have learned about meal timing and frequency of eating. This diet is relatively easy to implement. Just pick one or two non-consecutive days of the week where you don't eat for 24 hours. You can generally eat for the other five or six days. But it is recommended that you eat healthy for the best results. Even though it seems counter-intuitive, you will still eat every day of the calendar. How does it work? Imagine you have decided to start your fast at 9 am on Monday.

You take your last meal on Monday morning before 9 am. You can then eat your next food on Tuesday morning after 9 am. During the fasting hours, you need to stay well hydrated. Drink plenty of water and other calorie-free beverages such as tea or coffee without sweetener or milk.

If you want to try the eat-stop-eat method, you need to choose the right fasting day. This will be an individual choice. First, you must decide whether you will fast for one or two days. You may find it easier to start with one day of fasting per week. When you get used to it, you can increase it to 2 days each week. Do not exceed the number of days listed. Some people find it easier to fast on weekends because they don't have to focus on work. Other people prefer to fast on weekdays to have interference that prevents them from thinking about food. You must determine your own preferences. Remember, if you choose to do two days of fasting, they cannot be consecutive. This would be too long a period of fasting. You may need to experiment to find the correct pattern for you.

Other Types of Intermittent Fasting

Although 24-hour intermittent fasting and 16:8 fasting are the 2 most popular types, there are many others. Here, we will take a closer look at five kinds of other fasting regimens that some people follow.

20:4 Fasting

20:4 fasting is sometimes called the Warrior Diet. It is one of the first diets to involve intermittent fasting. Popular thanks to Ori Hofmekler, an Israeli fitness expert, this diet involves eating one large meal during the night. This hefty meal takes place in a four-hour window to eat. For another 20 hours, only a tiny number of raw vegetables and edible fruits. The food choice for this diet must be healthy - similar to the paleo diet. They should be confused that it is not processed that does not contain artificial ingredients.

5:2 Fasting

This popular form of intermittent fasting consists of eating normally for five days each week. On the remaining two days, calories should be limited to 500 to 600. Sometimes called the fasting diet, Michael Mosley, a famous journalist, popularized this way of eating. Women are recommended not to exceed 500 calories during their fasting days. Men can eat 600 calories on their fasting days. You can choose which two days you prefer to fast. However, it is better if they are not consecutive. On those days, you can choose to eat one meal or two small meals. Many people prefer to eat two meals of 250/300 calories each.

36-Hour Fasting

A quick 36-hour plan means you'll fast for an entire day. Unlike the EAT-stop-eat method, you won't eat anything for the whole of the day. If, for example, you finish dinner at 7 pm7 pm on the first day, you won't take any food for the entire day 2.

You will not eat your next food until day 3 at 7 am7 am. This equates to 36 hours. There is some evidence to suggest that this type of fasting period can produce faster results. This could also be helpful for diabetics, while it may be more problematic to manage and implement because you will be going for an extended period without food.

Alternate Day Fsting

Given the meaning of the term, fasting means that you don't have to take in calories for some time, usually lasting 24 hours or through alternative time schedules. Some of these versions of intermittent fasting allow you to eat up to 500 calories on the day you fast. Others only allow for calorie-free drinks. But this is definitely not the best choice for those who interface as a beginner to intermittent fasting. However, during the phase in which you fast, you go to sleep feeling hungry some nights during the week. Intermittent fasting is an effective, beneficial method but definitely complex to follow in the long run.

Extended Fasts

Following the 16:8 or eat-stop-eat method is pretty simple. However, some people want to encourage the maximum benefits of intermittent fasting. They prefer to even go as far as 42 hours of fasting! If you decide to test this method, you shouldn't limit your calorie intake during the meal window. However, it is possible to extend the fast for an even more extended period. In fact, the world record is 382 days. Of course, it is not recommended to follow this example!

Some people try fasting for 7 to 14 days because of the theoretical benefits listed. Some say that fasting can help prevent cancer. Others say that more extended fasting increases mental clarity, but this benefit is unproven and speculative. In any case, before approaching any of the intermittent fasting methods listed and described in this text, it is a must to consult an experienced nutritionist or dietitian who will follow you and establish the best plan for your needs.

How to get Started with Intermittent Fasting

If you are confident in the benefit of intermittent fasting, you need to know how to get started. However, starting any new regimen can be complicated. So, how can you get started in the best way possible? Here are some of the best tips.

Starting with a less Rigorous Regime

It might be tempting to try to lose as much weight as possible by starting quickly. However, remember that this may not be the best approach. As we mentioned, it may be difficult to fast for a long time if you've never done it before. If you are familiar with a high-carb, high-sugar, processed food diet, you will altogether avoid fasting for 36 hours. It is recommended that you try the intermittent fasting plan for at least a month. This time will be necessary to understand if intermittent fasting is proper for you and how you can adapt it according to your needs. It will be challenging for someone with no experience to stay on the intermittent fasting regimen for the long term. Therefore, those who are starting out should choose the less strict regimens, to begin with.

The 5: 2 diet allows you to eat food every day. In fact, you can eat your usual food five days a week. The other two days, you will have to stick to the 500-calorie regimen. This will give you many choices, as long as you make a healthy choice. Choose your food wisely, and you will experience the benefits without feeling hungry. Or try the 16:8 method, which is very popular.

Consider that for most of the time you are fasting, you will be sleeping. You will be free to eat whatever you want (reasonably) during your 8-hour meal window. Many people like the freedom offered by this pattern. When they are used to fasting for 16 consecutive hours, they find this eating relatively easy. If you want to work up to a longer fast once you get used to the fast, you can. However, many people follow their original plan in the long term and get good results.

Staying Hydrated

Regardless of what type of fasting routine you apply, you need to be well hydrated. Fasting is implemented by avoiding calorie-dense foods and drinks. This does not mean you can't drink water or other calorie-free beverages. In fact, you need to drink more! Staying hydrated ensures that toxins are effectively removed from your body. This will help you carry out your weight loss goals and maintain good health. This can help you take care of your health in other ways as well. Your skin will become healthier, toned, glowing, and younger-looking. Also, your bowel habits will be more regular. You will also avoid headaches and other problems related to dehydration. Drinking no-calorie drinks while fasting can also help keep you from feeling hungry. We often think we are hungry, but we are actually thirsty. If you drink a glass of water when you feel hungry, you will starve longer.

Try Experimenting with Different Eating Patterns

I have suggested some of the diet plans above, but that doesn't mean that you should necessarily stick to them. The days and times I offer are just examples. They may not work for everyone. You need to choose the right day and diet that fits your lifestyle, preferences, and needs. You may want to start eating as soon as you wake up and eat your last meal early. Or you may want to stop hunger pangs in the afternoon and have one last meal before bed. You may want to fast on the weekends, so you don't have to worry about feeling tired at work. Or fasting on a weekday might be just the thing to take your mind off things. No Intermittent fasting package is perfect for everyone. That means you may need to do some experimenting. Weigh the pros and cons of each of the modes you now know. Think about which one may be more appealing to you and give it a try. It's best to give yourself a month to see if it works for you. If you encounter problems, it's time to go back to the drawing board. Try another regular fast to see if it's more compatible with your lifestyle. Or move your lunch window slightly to see if it's easier to work with. Don't be afraid to experiment - in the end, experimentation can be the key to success.

Remember to always consult with a specialist who will follow your journey step by step while also assessing your body's response to this significant change in eating habits.

What Can You Eat and Drink While Intermittent Fasting

Should You Watch Your Diet? Indeed, regardless of whether you participate in a regular fasting program, you should always pay attention to what you are eating. The number one cause of health problems, disease, and obesity is the food we eat. In fact, deep in our hearts, we know what to eat. Vegetables and fruits are necessary for good health. They are full of vitamins, minerals, antioxidants, and fiber. The human body craves vegetables. However, our current diet is more focused on processed meat. There is only a tiny portion of volatile vegetables, which in many cases do more harm than good. French fries, eggplant and peppers in oil, and mashed potatoes in gravy are not vegetables. Vegetables are defined as broccoli, cabbage, celery, cucumbers, kale, and many other varieties. Sometimes vegetables don't satisfy our taste buds. If they aren't made palatable with a few tricks, it could be bored to eat them. However, they are very beneficial for your health. Getting into the habit of eating vegetables can help you in the long run. Vegetables are essential in regular fasting.

You can eat more vegetables and keep your calorie count down because vegetables usually contain fewer calories. They are also more satiating, as they are rich in fiber and are less likely to make you hungry during the fasting window. The same goes for fruits. Eat a wide variety of fruit and make sure it's 100% natural. Always eat fruit instead of just drinking juice packs. Fiber keeps your body good and insulin levels stable. Avoid processed fruit that comes in cardboard boxes. Commercial fruit juices should also be avoided because they are full of additives and added sugar, both of which are dangerous substances for your health. In addition to vegetables, you need to get protein from healthy cuts of meat—cook meat in a healthy way by roasting or steaming it. You can boil meat if you like. Fried and processed meats such as sausages and frankfurters should be avoided or consumed at a minimum. They are high in calories and preservatives and very fatty. In addition to meat protein and plant-based carbohydrates, you also need healthy fats. There are 2 amazing sources of healthy fats: extra virgin olive oil and raw coconut oil. Coconut oil is very beneficial. In the past, it had a bad reputation for causing high cholesterol. However, recent research has shown that this was just a false myth; coconut oil is actually perfect for health. Anyway, I suggest you do your research on nutrition and read up on what foods are best to consume for your needs. They are highly beneficial to our bodies and fight to age. Choosing healthy food will serve us to improve body functions, keep us healthy, rejuvenate and eliminate free radicals. However, regarding intermittent fasting, it has been proven that you could safely lose weight even by eating junk food in the window dedicated to the activity of eating. This is as long as you remain in a caloric deficit. However, your goal is to lose weight and stay healthy. Weight loss is only a consequence of a healthy and robust physique. The best way to stay healthy is to eat healthily. All the sports in the world will not make you healthy if you have a terrible diet. You can be weak and fit, but if the food you eat is unhealthy, you will have health problems sooner or later. Gradually eliminate your bad food choices and replace them with healthier ones. For example, replace hydrogenated oil with coconut oil. Or replace orange juice bought at your grocery store with fresh oranges.

Every little change helps. Once your diet is proper, and you stick to the intermittent fasting plan, you become a fat-burning machine. You will lose fat faster, and you will also feel more energetic and generally feel better. You will not be able to explain it. Your mood will improve. You will feel more alive, and life as a whole will seem much better. You will be surprised that the clouds that have covered you for a long time seem to have lifted. That is the power of a clean diet.

Unhealthy Foods You Should Remove from Your Diet

When someone hear the word diet, they usually think of a transient eating situation that allows them to gain or lose weight. This could not be further from the truth. The word diet describes how you eat in general because you have a generally healthy or unhealthy diet. Since people tend to get confused when they talk about diet changes, I like to call them lifestyle changes. Suppose you truly intend to lose weight and become a generally healthier person. In that case, once you've lost the amount of weight you wanted, you can't rely on dieting for a while and then go back to your regular eating habits. You don't. What you're going to do is employ your efforts to lose weight and do the same afterward to continue eating healthy, beneficial foods. The only way to change your figure and maintain it, in the long run, is to change your lifestyle in the long run. The most crucial aspect of your lifestyle is your diet: what you eat. Once you understand what you need to be healthy, stick to diet assiduously to continue to reap the benefits of a given eating style. Find an ideal manner and maintain it for the rest of your life. Negligent dieting will only increase your negative dieting experiences!

Let's get the not-so-fun part out of the way first. There are foods you should avoid eating altogether; personally, I don't recommend taking them even in moderation. Fortunately for many of you, this list is short. However, almost anything sweet and tasty can be part of your new diet if consumed in moderation.

Trans-Fats

There are so many reasons why this type of fat should be excluded entirely from the diet. There is really no good reason to eat them. They have no health benefits and are very dangerous. Even by common nutrition standards, trans-fats are at the bottom of the food pyramid. As an essential nutrient, it would be very regrettable to be associated with trans fats if fat could speak. The sneaky thing about trans fats is that food companies can say they are not contained within the product if their amount is below a specific value. Read the nutrition labels and ingredients of the products you buy carefully. This will almost always tell you if there is a small number of trans fats.

Such small amounts may not be dangerous, but still, avoid buying from these companies. It might be an excellent suggestion to avoid them altogether.

High-Sugar Energy Drinks

I know this is the hardest part to get rid of. Many people really love this intense energy drink. And why wouldn't they? Not only is it bursting with sugar and flavor, but it's also wholly decided thanks to caffeine, an addictive substance! You might think caffeine is harmless and inoffensive because it's found in many drinks, from coffee to soda, but like many illegal drugs, but caffeine is addictive.

The company that makes energy drinks puts tons of sugar in then adds large amounts of caffeine. When they reached the legal limit for caffeine, they used a similar type: guarana seed extract. This extract is basically just more caffeine; however, because it's made from the seeds and the process is different from adding caffeine to a drink, you could exceed the maximum allowable dosage this way. In fact, when you drink this energy drink, you may be drinking more than the legal, safe limit for caffeine. Caffeine is a powerful stimulant that can keep you awake. It can also cause panic attacks, high blood pressure, paranoia, or heart attacks in large doses!

And the terrible thing about this drink is that it's full of stimulants and sugar. Although you can get energy from it, the disaster you get when you're ready to store all that sugar can knock you out! If you can find a low-sugar energy drink with moderate caffeine content, then go for it. Still, I honestly recommend avoiding these things altogether. The main thing is always to use your common sense.

Things to Keep in Moderation

The absolute key to success when approaching any good diet plan is moderation. We are surrounded by millions of tasty foods, and it would be a massive shame if we had to give up these treats every day of our lives and only force ourselves to eat what is good for us. Who doesn't want to enjoy a delicious piece of chocolate cake or a well-toasted slice of bread topped with butter and jam?

Anyway, eating treats and tasty food every now and then can be part of a healthy lifestyle, plus this food helps relieve tension and acts as a reward. You just have to make sure that the approach to these foods is not a habit but something sporadic. Eating a wonderful slice of chocolate cake on the weekend is fine; eating one a day means waiting for a heart attack! Moderating your intake of unhealthy foods will not only improve your health and lose weight, but it will also make those foods even more special. You'll find that your favourite comfort food tastes even better when you've been waiting all week to get some.

On the other hand, you may find that some of your old favourite foods no longer appeal to you after you start eating healthy. Also, many people on low-fat diets tend to get sick more quickly when they replenish these fats in their diets; the body can't always handle sudden changes in diet as well as it can, so I recommend that you take extra care with your food management.

Anti-aging Superfoods

Following a proper diet and healthy lifestyle helps you stay young longer and age well. As mentioned above, the skin is the largest organ in our body. It represents one of the most critical barriers to our body. First of all, in fact, it has to fight against ultraviolet radiation, chemical agents, various pollutants and at the same time has the thankless task of eliminating many of the toxic substances introduced into our body. This exhausting work, over the years, inevitably leaves marks on the skin, some of the most common skin manifestations such as furrows and wrinkles, more or less pronounced, and the appearance of skin spots and dyschromia. The protection of the skin, therefore, does not only come from the outside, that is, from the application of moisturizers and protective or soothing masks, but also, and perhaps above all, from the inside, from what we eat every day and the behaviors we put in place every day at the table.

It has been scientifically proven that eating habits and the foods we consume play a vital role in slowing down or accelerating the aging process. You have undoubtedly experienced the damaging effects on your skin of an unbalanced diet. Dry or oily skin, pimples, and blackheads, loss of shine, accumulation of impurities are just some of the consequences of an unbalanced and wrong diet. Paying more attention to what we eat, and drink will allow us to properly fight the signs of aging while maintaining healthy, toned, and shiny skin. An incorrect diet, rich in sugars and fats, contributes to premature aging that involves the outward appearance and the entire body.

Instead, eating well and less helps the organism slow down the natural aging process and allows it to age better, giving a chance of longevity to one's prospects of life. To a correct and balanced diet, we must not forget to also associate a healthy lifestyle. This means doing movement and adequate physical activity even at home, drinking plenty of water for good hydration, and in general, adopting healthy behaviors in every field.

With a healthy and balanced diet, favoring foods rich in antioxidants such as vitamins A, C, E, beta-carotene, lycopene, lutein, we can fight free radicals. Foods that help to stay young should, therefore, be considered and encouraged.

What are free radicals?

Free radicals are responsible for skin aging, sagging skin tissue, and the appearance of wrinkles. But also, pathologies such as arthritis and arthrosis, dermatitis, chronic bronchitis, and asthma. The action of free radicals can affect the proper functioning of cardiovascular system. It can cause diabetes, pulmonary emphysema, cataracts, and Parkinson's and Alzheimer's diseases.

The role of omega 3

Among the anti-aging foods, there are essential fatty acids, good fats contained mainly in fish, and ideal for keeping cholesterol at bay and keeping the walls of the veins elastic. Moreover, they fight the action of free radicals. Like other fats, they facilitate the absorption of fat-soluble vitamins such as A, D, E, and K, which have an anti-aging effect. They also stimulate metabolism, increasing its efficiency, especially in burning fats and carbohydrates. But how can aging be slowed down with food?

The answer is given by science. In recent years, applied research has made it possible to identify a series of foods containing nutrients and active ingredients that help protect the skin from the signs of aging. These foods, defined as superfoods, hide within them a series of substances defined as nutraceuticals, capable of exerting a real anti-aging action. It is necessary to know the anti-aging foods, in short, foods rich in antioxidants to stay in perfect health and maintain a good appearance. And have young and wrinkle-free skin! There are metabolic areas in the body that actively participate in aging process through natural chemical reactions with the substances of which the foods we eat are composed. This is why, for example, it is so important to consume foods rich in antioxidants and anti-inflammatory substances such as fruits, vegetables, and whole grains.

They can decrease and slow down those fundamental processes that regulate the path of aging. This speech, moreover, assumes more excellent value if referred to women in menopause. In this delicate phase that every woman goes through between the ages of 45-55, metabolism tends to slow down, causing a progressive accumulation of fat. Keeping fit and preserving muscle mass, therefore, becomes essential not only to take care of one's own beauty but also to question the well-being of the organism and prevent premature aging.

The top experts in anti-aging medicine say that the best anti-aging diet includes a variety of foods rich in vitamins, natural substances such as zinc, magnesium, and potassium, as well as natural antioxidants, such as legumes and whole fiber, seasonal fruits and vegetables, but also fish and whole grains. Obviously, we are not talking about an elixir of eternal life. The aging of the cells of our body is a process impossible to stop. Still, with some corrections to eating habits (and a healthy lifestyle that includes physical activity and sports), you can slow down this phenomenon and, at the same time, age in a better way, with beautiful skin, toned and staying fit.

To stay young despite menopause, it is best to prefer simple and unprocessed foods, avoiding excessive consumption of foods rich in sugar, refined grains such as pasta, packaged foods, and overly salty foods such as fried foods, meats, and chocolate. Young skin comes by eating.

According to a ground-breaking study from the University of Cambridge, you can reduce wrinkles and change your appearance through the diet alone. From the latest scientific research, here's a guide to the "superfoods" that make your skin look good and help keep it young.

So here is a list of SUPERFOODS to include in your anti-aging diet and some advice for a more conscious and healthy diet, especially suitable for women over 40, 50, and 60 in menopause.

Almonds

Reduce damage produced by free radicals due to the presence of vitamin E. Almonds contain protein, iron, zinc. They are highly energetic and, at the same time, easily digestible. Almonds have a high caloric content (600 kcal/100gr), so it is necessary not to exceed the quantities. They are rich in monounsaturated and polyunsaturated fatty acids, essential for cardiovascular protection. Thanks to the presence of fibers, if consumed regularly, they facilitate the natural intestinal transit.

Flax seeds and chia seeds

Excellent source not only of fibers, essential to preserve the intestinal integrity and the absorption of other nutrients but especially of alpha-linolenic acid, essential fatty acid of the omega 3 series, endowed with a marked anti-inflammatory activity.

Whole Grains

Choose whole grains over refined grains because they have more fiber, vitamins, minerals, and essential fatty acids, making them ideal for the heart and gut health. Numerous foods fall into this category. From classic whole grains, such as pearl rice and wheat, to lesser consumed grains such as spelt, barley, quinoa, and oats. You can consume whole grains in about half of your meals each day. For example, if you eat whole grain bread for breakfast, you can have white rice or something else of your choice for lunch.

Goji berries, carrots, mangoes, apricots, pumpkin

Valuable resources of beta-carotene, a pigment proven to be even more potent than vitamin E in protecting skin structures from damage induced by ultraviolet radiation.

Tomato

Made up of almost 95% water, tomato is rich in minerals and antioxidants such as lycopene, beta-carotene (vitamin A), and vitamin C. A powerful ally to fight to age. Just lycopene, contained in tomatoes, is one of the most potent antioxidants present in nature. It protects against lipid peroxidation and LDL (the "bad" cholesterol). It also helps the body fight cardiovascular disease among the best anti-aging foods.

Oily fish: Fish is the food richest in minerals, lean protein, and anti-inflammatory Omega 3 acids. For this reason, the consumption of fish - preferably oily fish (salmon, cod, sardine, mackerel) - should be repeated at least two or three times a week. It is better to avoid eating big fish such as tuna or swordfish. Instead, prefer local, more nutritious, and cheaper.

Pomegranate

The juice obtained from pomegranate is a rich source of antioxidants, which are good in fighting the appearance of free radicals. Pomegranate contains several minerals, such as calcium, magnesium, potassium, copper, sulfur, phosphorus, and iron. It has astringent and diuretic properties. Among the best and most known characteristics is the anti-aging one.

Red Grapes

It contain many minerals (iron, calcium, phosphorus, sodium, and magnesium). It is a fruit rich in boron, a trace element that promotes the assimilation of calcium and its deposition in bone tissue. Thanks to resveratrol, it protects from cardiovascular diseases and has anti-inflammatory, antioxidant action. It contrasts the production of free radicals, promotes skin tonicity, and stimulates the production of collagen.

Walnuts: Walnuts and, in general, dried fruits are the ideal hunger breaker snack to be consumed before a fitness session to give the body the right amount of energy. These foods enjoy numerous properties helpful in slowing down the aging process. They contain large amounts of vitamins, antioxidants, and healthy fatty acids. Eating a handful of almonds/walnuts at snack time is a good energy recharge that quenches the sense of hunger while helping you healthily lose weight. Also, walnuts are an excellent source of minerals and fiber, have anti-inflammatory properties, and help fight hypercholesterolemia, improving the functioning of the digestive system and immune system. Recent studies have shown that consuming 3-4 nuts a day (or other dried fruits) benefits our cardiovascular system due to their unsaturated fatty acids, magnesium, and fiber content. Rich in polyphenols, powerful antioxidants, they help prevent the diseases of aging. They are rich in vitamin E, an essential nutrient for the prevention of dementia. Three nuts a day positively affect our health. Brazil nuts also have a very high selenium content, the anti-aging mineral par excellence: two nuts contain our daily requirement. Recent studies have shown that the regular and daily consumption of nuts can also prevent prostate cancer. Greenlight then to two Brazil nuts a day!

Blueberries

Anthocyanosides (blue, red, purple pigments found in the plant kingdom) contained in blueberries boast necessary antioxidant power, which limits cellular aging. They are foods that help to stay young. Blueberries, which are very rich in vitamin C, fiber, also have remarkable healing powers. It fights visual fatigue because it stimulates the production of rhodopsin. It improves the ability to see in low light conditions. It also fortifies the wall of capillary vessels, fighting fragility and the vascular permeability, and helps against intestinal disorders.

Turmeric

Besides being a powerful ally for our brain, turmeric is a powerful anti-inflammatory very useful in arthritis. Use it often to flavor all dishes: just a pinch if you use turmeric powder or a few gills if you use a fresh one, even more, effective than powdered.

Soy

This natural ingredient has a high concentration of isoflavones. They promote female well-being and help reduce cholesterol and fight cardiovascular disease.

Cruciferous vegetables

This category includes Brussels sprouts, cauliflower, turnips, broccoli, and cabbage. They are rich in polyphenols, substances that help the body cleanse itself, promoting toxin elimination and detoxification. They are cruciferous because of the shape all the vegetables belonging to this family take, that is, with four petals flowers arranged in a cross shape.

Pineapple

Fresh pineapple is the only known source of "bromelain," an enzyme that helps our bodies absorb protein. It is effective in reducing inflammation, relieving joint and muscle pain. It is also a natural anticoagulant. It should be consumed at least 2 times a week.

Beets

Rich in vitamin E and K, they fight free radicals. Due to the presence of folic acid and betalains (the pigments that make them colorful), they are powerful antioxidants. They also contain vitamins A, C, B, PP, copper, phosphorus, zinc, calcium, potassium, and chlorophyll. They are rich in minerals and trace elements.

Salmon

Salmon is rich in Omega-3 fats that play a crucial role in protecting and repairing cell membranes. Omega-3 fats also keep blood pressure and triglyceride levels regular and help skin stay hydrated, preventing the appearance of wrinkles. Just 2 servings per week are enough to benefit from its nutritional properties.

Avocado

Avocado is an exotic fruit that appears more and more often on the tables of many people. Avocado is among the seven anti-aging foods due to its large dose of healthy monounsaturated fats, antioxidants, and protective phytonutrients. In other words, including avocado in your diet will help you prevent skin aging, being rich in vitamins A and E, and protect the health of your heart and blood vessels. Beware of excess, though. Avocados are also high in calories, so I recommend consuming them no more than twice a week.

Spinach

They are vegetables with the highest iron content, rich in vitamins E and K.
If consumed regularly, they are good allies in the fight against free radicals and aging. They also provide a good dose of calcium, phosphorus, and magnesium. They also have laxative, antianemic, and antioxidant properties thanks to the carotenoids, folic acid, chlorophyll, and lutein. Rich in alpha-lipoic acid and vitamins, they counteract the structural damage produced by oxygen free radicals towards the structures of the dermis.

Beans

As far as anti-aging foods go, beans are among the best around (e.g., organic Adzuki green beans). Your heart will love the healthy, fat-free protein, as well as the other anti-aging properties of beans. Beans are an excellent anti-aging and longevity food. They provide healthy protein without all (unhealthy) fats found in animal products. Beans also offer many antioxidants that prevent free radical damage. Incorporate the anti-aging properties of beans into your weekly menu.

Raspberries

Raspberries are an essential source of manganese, a mineral that can increases bone density. Consume 2 servings per week to prevent osteoporosis.

Arugula

Arugula helps reduce blood pressure and is a good source of folate (vitamin B9 folic acid), which helps prevent anemia. It is essential for the formation of hemoglobin. Include it at least 2 times a week in your diet.

Ginger

Ginger is food with countless properties that offer several benefits to the body. The "health root," ginger, has a powerful anti-inflammatory and an antioxidant effect that makes it valuable against digestive disorders. The best choice to enjoy its beneficial effects is to consume it in herbal teas and infusions.

Berries

The raspberries, blueberries, and blackberries are rich in vitamins and antioxidants, counteract the action of free radicals and promote blood circulation. Rich in lycopene (a pigment), it has been shown effective not only in strengthening skin's antioxidant defenses but also in controlling the synthesis of proteins in the dermis and inhibiting the proliferation of malignant cells.

Dark Chocolate

Dark chocolate is rich in tannins and flavonoids, known antioxidants, which protect the cardiovascular system and help the body prevent the formation of free radicals, delaying their harmful action. Dark chocolate also provides potassium, magnesium, theobromine, a substance that gives an energy boost. It contains procyanidin, which has a protective action against cancer degeneration. Dark chocolate has anti-aging properties, and this is proof that the universe is a loving, unique, and kind place. Eat a little chocolate every day after lunch to enjoy its anti-aging benefits (don't overdo it, of course, it can be irritating). Choose organic and artisanal ones, preferably. It is one of the most appreciated foods in the world. Recent research shows that eating moderate amounts of dark chocolate also benefits heart health. The antioxidants in dark chocolate protect the heart from aging and heart disease. But make sure it's at least 70% dark chocolate. Avoid like the plague industrial fake milk chocolate or the other super sugary chocolate.

Green Tea

It is a valuable ancient beverage for health and longevity; Chinese and Japanese know this very well. The antioxidant benefits of green tea consumption are well known. A small amount of green tea (the organic kind) a couple of times a day could do wonders for your life expectancy. Drink green tea with meals, it will feel strange at first, but once you get used to it, you won't be able to do without it (don't drink it cold!).

Ensure it's a natural organic green tea; the industrial bagged ones equate to drinking nothing or pesticides.

Red wine

Good news for wine lovers! Red wine has properties that make you look younger. Just one glass a day has incredible anti-aging benefits (one glass of wine a day, not 5!). Red wine has been found to offer a multitude of health benefits. In fact, more than 400 scientific studies support the claim of the services that red wine can provide. Always choose to drink organic wine. Otherwise, you will also be ingesting pesticides.

Water

Our bodies need water to fight aging and the damage we cause. Drink plenty of water every day to keep your body functioning well. Water can be healthy and "detoxifying" for your body. But beyond that, drinking plenty of water is a good thing because it keeps you busy by preventing you from drinking other sugary, industrial beverages.

So, in addition to protecting your skin from the outside, try to take these little precautions so that you will always be young and glowing! The consumption of these foods helps reduce the risks of chronic diseases, reducing inflammation, and promoting lower blood pressure. Anti-aging nutrition is also part of a beauty routine. In fact, beautiful skin can be achieved (even) at the table thanks to foods that reduce wrinkles and ward off aging.

How To Track Your Nutrition Intake Easily and Effectively

Just exercising and not having good nutrition doesn't guarantee you will lose weight, build muscle or perform at your best. I often talk to people who want them to work out but aren't getting the results they want. I find that there is nothing particularly wrong with what they are doing in the gym. Still, they are not seeing results because they are not supporting their efforts with good nutrition. For weight loss, you need to make sure you have a sufficient and sustainable calorie deficit.

Monitoring your food intake will give you a clear picture of what is entering your body in the form of nutrients. This means you'll be able to make better choices and see the best results from your workouts. It's worth it to learn how to fuel your body so that you get the best out of it, feel your best, and make it last as long as possible. I understand that nutrition tracking can seem like a bit of a pain, so now, I'm going to simplify this process for you right here, right now. Let's go.

How to track your nutrition

You can try many websites or download apps on your mobile phone about it. Many of them are free, easy to use, and have a lot of valuable features. The best ones are also used by most fitness professionals and athletes I know. Do some research, and make sure you download a professional and comprehensive app. Once you've found it, you can proceed with entering your information:

Create an account, enter your parameters (weight, height, age, etc.), and your goals: lose/maintain/increase weight. The app uses this kind of information to estimate a daily calorie goal for you. It also provide you with some predefined macronutrient goals to aim for. Macronutrients are carbohydrates, fats, and proteins. So, you need an ideal balance of these macronutrients to see the results you're looking for.

I highly recommend that you have a professional calculate your calorie and macronutrient goals for you, as they will be able to take your individuality into consideration and adjust your goals over time based on your progress. Alternatively, you can calculate your calorie and macronutrient goals yourself. Either way, it's easy to set tailored goals in the app. Sometimes apps allow you to enter information about your physical activity. If your goal is to lose weight, I recommend not using this feature. It will increase your calorie quota for the day, which could affect how quickly you lose weight. Simply consider the calories burned through exercise as a bonus. If you're looking to gain muscle or your goal is athletic performance, this feature is more relevant. However, your activity level should have already been considered when your calorie goals were initially calculated. The most ideal way to monitor your food intake would be to stick to "real" foods (i.e., meat, vegetables, grains, fruits, etc.), measuring amounts by eye. Whatever your goal is, here's an excellent general guide:

Keep track of your food intake in detail for quite a few weeks at first. This will allow you to gather enough data to consider your findings reliable. It will also help you start to build a framework of what your ideal diet will look like. Over time, you'll become more able to eat intuitively without relying on food tracking apps to know that you've given your body everything it needs - no more, no less. Track your intake for each day of the week.

A common mistake is to only track weekdays and end up having absolutely no idea what you ate on the weekends. For example, a higher calorie intake on the weekend could completely ruin your weekday efforts to maintain a healthy calorie deficit. After this initial period, keep track for a week to make sure you are still on target. It is essential that even when you're not tracking, you're making a conscious effort to continue making the best nutritional decisions possible. It can be all too easy to give up good habits when there is no data to record to keep you accountable! Once you've reached your goal, go back to consistently monitoring for a short period so that you can figure out how to maintain your weight loss/muscle gain/recovery from your sports competition. You will benefit from doing this during any transition period, whether it's reaching a weight loss goal or entering menopause. Know that nothing ever stays the same, and your needs are constantly changing.

How to analyze your nutritional data

You can monitor your intake daily, but I find it more helpful to look at your data one week at a time. This can help many people avoid food obsession. Evaluate how many calories you eat per day and overall, each week. Are you eating too much or too little? If so, how often? Check how much your macronutrient intake is in line with your goals. Start noticing trends: the days of the week when you are more or less successful in reaching your goals and figure out why.

Play around with the app and learn about the content of the different kinds of foods you eat. Identify the foods and meals that provide you with the best calorie and macro balance so you can make them more often. Identify foods or meals that hinder your progress and try to reduce the frequency with which you eat them. If you've taken notes in the app, you can also evaluate how different foods make you feel and affect your performance. Always consider your training in line with your nutrition: how does your diet affect your progress toward your goals?

You'll never achieve total accuracy...and that's okay! It's better to have approximate data than no data at all. My best advice here would be to link your new food tracking habit to an existing one. Always keep your priorities in mind. Remind yourself why you're monitoring, why it's essential, and what you're getting out of it. Rather than stressing over how much of a chore it is, train your brain to focus on the positive aspects. Looking at the data you collect and drawing conclusions can be a lot of fun. Remember to congratulate yourself on even the slightest progress.

Nutrition tracking can be easy and stay fun if you focus on building good habits, keeping priorities in the front of your eyes, and enjoying the learning process.

Suppose you are suffering because of an eating disorder or a history of disordered eating. In that case, nutrition monitoring could trigger problems for you. On the other hand, it could give you the information you need to fuel your body rather than deprive it of food. If you have this type of history, talk to a therapist, and start healing, my friend. Suppose you have accurately and realistically calculated your nutritional needs. In that case, you should never feel deprived of food or mainly restricted.

Just know that it takes a long time to change your eating habits, so take things day by day. I'm not demanding that people instantly abandon their current eating habits in favor of new ones. It's about making minor adjustments over time to improve your diet. If the process seems too intense, you could simply monitor your food and leave the data analysis to a professional, such as a qualified exercise coach or nutritionist. They can periodically review your results and suggest improvements you can make to your diet.

It all comes down to intention and mindset: are you ready and able to be kind to your body and yourself, give it what it needs, and not beat yourself up when you make mistakes?

Incorporating Exercise into Your Fasting Regime

Some research shows that if you exercise while fasting, there are additional benefits. There is an impact on your metabolism and muscle biochemistry. This is related to your insulin sensitivity and blood sugar levels. If you exercise during the fasting window, your glycogen (or stored carbohydrates) is depleted. This means you will burn more fat. For best results, eat protein after your workout. This will build and maintain your muscles. It will also promote better recovery. You should also eat carbohydrates within half an hour following an endurance workout.

It is wise to eat food close to any high-intensity exercise session or any exercise session. You should also drink a lot more water to stay well hydrated. Maintaining electrolyte levels is essential. Coconut water can be helpful for this. You may feel a little lightheaded or confused if you work out on an empty stomach. If you experience this discomfort, take a break. It is essential to listen to your body. If you are doing a longer fast, you may find that you can find light exercises such as Pilates, yoga, or walking are better. They help burn fat without making you feel sick.

So, should you exercise while fasting? As mentioned before, yes...you should definitely do it. There are many benefits of exercise such as:

- A higher metabolic rate which helps in fat loss

- Releases endorphins that make you feel happier

- Prevents muscle atrophy.

- Improves blood circulation

- Prevents diseases that cause cognitive decline

- Promotes better sleep

- Keeps your weight in check, and much more!

It may take a Herculean effort to make the transition from a sedentary lifestyle to an active one. The key here is minor, daily improvements. If you haven't exercised in years, you can start with 20 minutes of walking a day. So, should you exercise while fasting? As mentioned before, yes...you should definitely do it.

Don't jump into a high-intensity workout from one day to the next. Give your body time to adapt and recover. Start with low-impact exercises like walking, biking, and swimming. Then move on to resistance training with light weights. There is no need to train yourself to exhaustion when you're just starting out. The important thing is that you move more and get into the habit of exercising regularly. Over time, you can increase the intensity of your workouts and challenge yourself.

Keep in mind that it's okay to work out on an empty stomach. Still, you should have a meal within 45 minutes of completing your training. So, you could work out during your food window or start your food window after your workout.

That pretty much sums it up. A clean diet, intermittent fasting? And regular exercise is the three sides of the weight loss triangle. When you have all three components in place, you can lose weight, get healthier and fitter, and keep the excess pounds off. Many people live their lives like animals in a cage. Built to move, we too often confine ourselves. We have bodies designed to run across savannahs. Still, we live a lifestyle designed to migrate from bed to table, go to the car seat, and then to the office chair. At mealtime, we go to the restaurant booth, the living room couch, and back to bed. Repeat!

It hasn't always been that way. Not so long ago in the United States, a man working on a farm did the equivalent of 15 miles of jogging each day; and his wife did the same of 8 miles of jogging. Today, our daily habits keep us tied to our chairs, and if we want to exercise, we must seek it out. In fact, health experts insist that obesity is probably caused at least as much by a lack of physical activity as by overeating. So, it's essential that people need to get moving. However, that doesn't mean a lap or two around the old high school track will make up for a daily dose of donuts. Exercise alone is not very effective, experts say. They claim that if you just exercise and don't change your diet, you will prevent weight gain or lose a few pounds for a while.

However, that's not something you can sustain unless exercise is part of an overall program. The more regularly you exercise, the easier it is to maintain your weight. Here's what to do each day to make sure you're getting the exercise you need.

1. Get quality Zzzs

Make sure that you get adequate sleep. Good sleep habits are conducive to exercise, experts point out. If you feel worn out during the day, you are less likely to get much physical activity during the day. In addition, there is evidence that people who are tired tend to eat more, using food as a substance for the rest they need.

2. Walk the walk

It is probably the easiest exercise program of all. In fact, it may be all you ever have to do, according to some professional advices of some health experts. Gradually build up to at least 30 minutes of brisk walking five times a week. Brisk walks themselves have health and psychological benefits that are well worth the while.

3. Walk the treadmill

When the weather is bad, you might not feel like going outdoors. But if you have a treadmill in the television room, you can catch up on your favorite shows while you are doing your daily good turn for your weight-maintenance plan. Most of us watch television anyway, and indoor exercise equipment enables anyone to turn a sedentary activity into a healthy walk.

4. Seize the time.

Excuses aside, lack of time is certainly a limiting factor in most lifestyles. That is why health experts suggest a basic guideline for incorporating exercise into your schedule.

Get as much exercise as you can that feels good without letting it interfere with your work or family life. If you need to, remind yourself that you are preventing many health problems when you prevent weight gain; and keeping your health is a gift to your family as well as yourself.

The Final Healthy Lifestyle: How Losing Weight Triggers a Cascade of Health Benefits

There is an excellent benefit gained from losing weight. Although losing weight is not easy, long-term effects brought about by it would probably help anyone considering getting rid of those unwanted and unhealthy pounds. The following are some of the remarkable benefits of losing those excess pounds.

- **Weight loss prevents heart disease, high blood pressure, and stroke**

This is a 3-in-1 benefit of losing weight. It is an indisputable fact that heart disease and stroke are among the leading reasons for death in women and men in the United States and all over the World. Overweight people have a higher risk of having high cholesterol levels in their bloodstream and triglycerides (also known as blood fats). Angina, a heart disease, could cause chest pain and a decrease in oxygen pumped to the heart. Sudden death can also occur from stroke and heart disease, and usually, this hits with minimal warning, signs, and symptoms. It is a fact that is decreasing your weight by a mere five to ten percent could positively reduce your chances of having or developing heart disease or stroke. Also, the way your heart works would improve, and your blood pressure, cholesterol, triglycerides would decrease.

- **Weight loss prevents type 2 diabetes**

Diabetes endangers a person's life and the way they lead it because of complications that come with it. Both types of diabetes, type 1 and 2, are linked to being overweight. For those who already have diabetes, regular exercise and weight loss could help control blood sugar levels, as well as the medications you may currently be taking. Increase your physical activity. You could simply walk, jog or dance. It helps to get your bloodstreams moving and lose those unnecessary pounds.

- **Weight loss helps reduce cancer risk**

Being fat or overweight is linked with several types of cancer. Especially for women, common types of cancer associated with being fat include cancer of the uterus, gallbladder, ovaries, breast, and colon. I don't want to scare you but inform you. Also, men are at risk of developing cancer if they are fat. These include cancer of the prostate, colon, and rectum. Extra weight, a diet high in fat and cholesterol, should be avoided as much as possible.

- **Weight loss reduces or eliminates sleep apnea**

Sleep apnea is a condition in which you may temporarily stop breathing for a short time and then continue to snore heavily. Sleep apnea could also cause drowsiness during the day and - due to being overweight - could lead to heart failure. Getting rid of those excess pounds could help eliminate this problem.

- **Weight loss reduces osteoarthritis pain**

When a person weighs a lot, the joints in their knees, hips, and lower back have to exert twice - if not three times - as much effort to carry them throughout the day and when they exercise. This could cause strain and stress on these joints. Weight loss decreases the load these joints have, thus decreasing - if not eliminating - the pain of those with osteoarthritis.

I've given you a lot of information to think about. Now that you have the hard facts, you probably need to know what to do with them. We've discussed what you should eat, what you shouldn't eat, how you should exercise, and more about intermittent fasting after age 50. Now that you know which foods are good and evil, you need to make a complete lifestyle change about your diet. This is not a temporary thing to lose a few pounds. You have to create a routine that introduces variety but stays within your dietary requirements and is something you can continue until the end of your life. This is an absolute commitment; if you break the routine by going back to old bad habits, you will gain weight again. Promise yourself that you will never try another temporary diet again; there is no such thing as a quick diet being a good diet. I recommend that you try to balance when you eat your meals. Three times a day is the old gold standard, but I've heard of quite a few people who are much more successful by eating more frequently but with smaller meals. Instead of 3 large meals a day, eat 5 small meals. Another tactic you can employ is to have a large breakfast, a medium lunch, and a small dinner.

Breakfast should contain the most calories because it's fuelling you for the rest of the day; lunch can hold quite a few because you have half the day to work with, and dinner is the least important meal of all. What will you do after dinner besides relax and go to bed? Unless you eat dinner very early and party all night, there is no reason for it to be the most important meal of the day.

My final diet tip is to get the family involved. It is challenging to stick to a healthy diet when you are the only one doing it. You don't need a special, very low-calorie diet for yourself; if you stick to a healthy diet that would work for any individual, you will see results. Your diet should be good enough for everyone in your family (with some modifications for age).

Just as eating well is a lifelong commitment, so is physical activity. No matter how good your diet is, you'll gain the weight back if you don't keep exercising and working out. If you can't make a long-term commitment to a particular exercise or exercise program, then at least commit to an amount of time where you will be active every day and every week. Plan to do some form of physical activity or exercise for at least an hour every day (a minimum of 45 minutes a day). I find a happy and realistic medium for everyone to do 30 minutes of light exercise (like walking around your home) every day and 15 minutes of more intense workout (sprints or weightlifting) every day. Walk around your home in the morning and then lift 5- or 10-pound dumbbells before you go to bed. This will keep your metabolism up, build muscle and help you keep the extra weight off.

Don't give up!

Menopause is a compassionate time in a woman's life because profound physical and psychological changes occur during this period. One of the most frequent problems that afflict women is weight gain due to the reorganization of the hormonal balance, to which are added the slowing of the metabolism and attacks of nervous hunger as a result of the alteration of the mood.

Is it your goal to lose weight, but you feel like you can't? Don't be discouraged! Sure, losing weight during menopause may seem more difficult, but it's not impossible. The important thing is not to be in a hurry and not follow overly restrictive eating regimens to achieve rapid weight loss because they could be harmful.

Now I will provide you with some valuable tips to help you implement your remise en forme and not lose motivation.

First, do an honest analysis of your lifestyle. How? For example, by trying to answer questions like these: How much do you weigh? Do you eat a healthy diet? Do you exercise? Are you anxious or stressed?

Before implementing changes, you need to know that you have first and foremost a responsibility to take care of yourself and ensure your well-being. You can't succeed in losing weight the right way if you're not objective and accept that there are things to change. Also, be careful not to expect to get results too quickly - drastic weight loss can be detrimental. It takes gradualness, regularity, and consistency to get results. Once you figure out what aspects need to be changed, you can start working on yourself. I hope this advice has opened your eyes to some of your weight loss options. The most important lesson I have for you is to never give up.

On your journey to weight loss, you will encounter peaks and plateaus and even bounces a few times; losing weight is not an easy process. As long as you stick with it and realize that it is a long-term plan, you can succeed. The results are not instant; in fact, they are not fast at all. The point is that you are changing the way you live from here until the end, so if it takes a year or even if it takes five years, you are working towards a better person!

FAQ

When you're eager to start intermittent fasting, you'll want all the information you need at your fingertips. Although I have covered all the critical points throughout the chapters, there are essential questions to answer. Here we address some of the most common questions about intermittent fasting. I hope the answers help you make a final decision about whether Intermittent Fasting might be proper for you. It should also help you get started on your new lifestyle.

Exercise and fasting

Many people wonder if they can continue to exercise if they are fasting. In most cases, intermittent fasting will not prevent you from exercising long term. It just may take some time to adjust to the new regimen. Some people who follow this lifestyle even find they have more energy while fasting! Some people worry about losing muscle if they fast. However, it is possible to prevent this from happening. If you eat plenty of protein in your window and do regular resistance training, you will be fine. It may be a good idea to work out at the end of fasting period. Typically, you will feel hungry about 30 minutes after you finish your workout. If you break your fast at that time, you will feel satisfied.

What should you eat during your meal window?

When you follow an Intermittent Fasting lifestyle, there are no particular restrictions on what you can eat in your meal window. This is why intermittent fasting is different from other ways of dieting. You are not restricted to specific amounts or types of food. However, it is wise to remember that you should still make healthy choices. If you indulge too much regularly you will not see the benefits of Intermittent fasting. The best solution is to eat a balanced and healthy diet in your food window. This can help you maintain your energy while still losing weight. Foods that are nutrient-dense such as beans, nuts, whole grains, seeds, vegetables, and fruits, are always the best choices. You have to consume plenty of lean protein.

Some foods are especially beneficial if you follow this way of eating:

- Avocado - yes, it is very caloric. However, it is full of monounsaturated fats. This makes them very satiating. If you add half an avocado to your meal, you will feel much fuller.

- Fish - you should try to eat a minimum of 8 ounces of fish each week. Fish is high in healthy fats, protein, and vitamin D. Vitamin D is also suitable for brain health.

- Cruciferous vegetables - foods like cauliflower, Brussels sprouts, kale, and broccoli are great choices. They are high in fiber which helps you avoid constipation and feel fuller.

- Potatoes - many people worry that potatoes are rotten for you. However, they are delighted and will keep you full longer. You may prefer sweet potatoes, which have a lower sugar intake.

- Legumes, beans - although they are carbohydrates, they are low in calories and give you a lot of energy. Legumes and beans are also rich in fiber and protein.

- Probiotics - eating probiotic-rich foods like kefir and kombucha help keep your gut happy. This will help you avoid stomach problems when you're adjusting to this diet.

- Berries - strawberries, blueberries & others are full of nutrients like vitamin C. Berries are rich in flavonoids, known to speed up weight loss.

- Eggs - each egg has a whopping 6 grams of protein. Simple and quick to cook, eggs make you feel full.

- Walnuts - Yeah! walnuts are high in calories. However, walnuts are rich in polyunsaturated fats that help you feel full.

- Whole grains - yes, whole grains are carbs too! However, they are rich in fiber and protein. You don't need to eat too many of them to feel full for longer. Experts say that eating whole grains can increase your metabolism!

What can you eat in your fasting period?

So, you know what you can eat in your food window. What can you eat in your fasting period? The answer depends on which fasting you are doing. If you're doing the 5:2 diet, you can eat up to 500 calories on fasting days. Obviously, this is quite restrictive. So, you can Maximize the amount you can eat by including lots of low-calorie foods, high-nutrient foods. Vegetables and fruits are the key elements of your fasting days.

If you're doing one of the other fasting methods, you can't eat solid foods. You also cannot drink beverages that contain calories. Fortunately, though, there are many drinks you can drink to stay hydrated. It goes without saying that you should drink plenty of water in your fasting window. Both sparkling and still water is fine. If you wish, you can add a squeeze of lime or lemon for a little more flavor. You can also add some flavor with an orange slice or cucumber. However, you cannot add artificially sweetened enhancers. These may harm your fasting.

Another good drink for the fasting period is black coffee. It contains no calories and does not affect your insulin levels. You can choose from decaf or regular, but don't add sweeteners or milk. If you want more flavor, try adding spices like cinnamon. Some people say that black coffee may enhance the benefits of Intermittent fasting. Caffeine can support ketone production. It can also help support healthy blood sugar levels over the long term. A note of caution, though. Some people find that if they drink coffee while fasting, they experience stomach pain or a racing heartbeat. Constantly monitor how you feel while taking black coffee!

If you have been fasting for 24 hours or more, try vegetable or bone broth. However, do not use bouillon cubes or canned broth. It is full of preservatives and artificial flavors that will harm your fast. Make it at home for the best results.

Tea can also help you feel full. You can drink any kind of tea during your fasting window. Oolong, black, green, and herbal teas are all good. Tea also helps to enhance fasting by supporting cell and gut health and probiotic balance. Green tea is perfect for managing weight and helping you feel full.

Apple cider vinegar offers many health benefits. You can add it to the list of things you can eat during your fasting period. It will support your blood sugar levels and digestion. It may also Increase the results of your fasting. However, there are some drinks that you need to avoid while you are fasting. You may not realize that "zero-calorie" sodas can break your fast. While diet sodas technically have no calories, they have been shown to inhibit the positive effects of fasting. This is because they get their sweet taste from aspartame or other artificial sweeteners. These trigger your insulin response. Therefore, you should avoid drinking them in your fasting window.

Many people ask if they can drink coconut water or almond milk during the fasting period. While both are healthy options with benefits for your well-being, they contain a lot of sugar. Since sugar is a carbohydrate, you will no longer be fasting if you consume it. You should not drink these drinks during the fasting period.

A prevalent question is whether you can drink alcohol if you are on an IF diet. You must limit your alcohol consumption to your food window. This is because most alcoholic beverages contain many calories and a lot of sugar. Therefore, drinking them will break your fasting period. Obviously, alcohol will have more effect on you if you have an empty stomach. Even one glass of wine can make you feel sick!

Conclusion

The program of intermittent fasting is highly effective, safe, and sustainable. One of the most significant advantages of Intermittent fasting is that it can be adopted for a lifetime. Unlike a diet that only works for a short period, intermittent fasting is a lifestyle. You'll eat real food and get all the macronutrients you need. There are no particular restrictions. The fasting period will take care of the fat-burning process. Your body will also have more energy because it is not constantly digesting food. The insulin levels of your body will be more stable, and your insulin sensitivity will really improve. This will make you less likely to gain weight. If you are considering adopting intermittent fasting, you should definitely give it a try.

Stay focused and committed. It will be difficult at first, but nothing worth having ever comes easy. As long as you stay on top of it, you'll get used to it and won't be able to look back. Monitor your progress and how you feel. Write it all down in a journal. In a few weeks, you'll see that you've made a great decision by adopting intermittent fasting. Once you see the benefits, you can tell your friends and family about it and encourage them to join you.

"Instead of using a medication, rather, fast one day." - Plutarch.

Now you know everything about intermittent fasting. If you're ready to experiment, this book should tell you everything you need to know to get started.

Identify the reasons why you want to try intermittent fasting. You may want to lose weight or improve your health. Maybe you just want to see if it makes you feel more focused and energetic. If you know what benefits you'd like to know, you'll be in a better position to succeed. You'll also be able to prioritize the strategy and foods that will be best for your goals. As you've seen in this book, there are several Intermittent fasting plans to choose from.

You'll need to consider which one is right for you by talking to an expert who will be with you along the way. You might prefer a daily approach with something like the 16:8 diet. Alternatively, a weekly plan like alternate day fasting or the 5:2 might be right for you. You'll need to consider your schedule and personal preferences.

Think about the times you get up and go to bed. When do you tend to get hungry? How busy are you during your day? Do you work out? The answers to these questions are essential to help you choose your food window. If intermittent fasting is going to be successful for you, it must fit effectively into your lifestyle. You need to be sure you can maintain your diet long-term. You will only be able to do this if it fits your needs. Remember that intermittent fasting should make your life easier, not harder. If it is too difficult to follow, you will give up too quickly. You should try following the diet for a minimum of one month to see if it works for you. When you get intermittent fasting right, you should reap the benefits quickly. Not only should you lose weight, but you should feel more energetic, healthy, and strong. You'll feel more focused and experience a range of health, beauty and wellness benefits. From the reduced chance of developing diabetes to a potentially longer lifespan, the benefits are numerous. So, what are you waiting for? Now is the time to try intermittent fasting. You're sure to experience the benefits!